HOPE
in the
HEARTACHE

A Journey of Grace & Growth
with a Special Needs Child

Kelly Speck

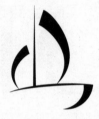

Ballast Books, LLC
Washington, DC
www.ballastbooks.com

ISBN 978-1-955026-11-6

Library of Congress Control Number has been applied for

Cover Designer: David Provolo
Photographer: Katie McMurry

Printed in Canada

Published by Ballast Books
www.ballastbooks.com

For more information, bulk orders, appearances or speaking requests,
please email info@ballastbooks.com

"Rejoice in hope, be patient in tribulation,
be constant in prayer."
— Romans 12:12

We dedicate this book to Bennett, Jackson and Reagan,
our three greatest gifts. May you hold tight
to HOPE when the winds of life blow;
and know that our love for you never waivers.

CONTENTS

INTRODUCTION

"It is like your newborn son is drowning. His lungs are filled with pneumonia. We do not believe he will survive."

As the petite young NICU fellow uttered these words to two stunned first-time parents, a deep pain shot into our bodies and set up camp. Blood gases. Organs shutting down. After a near-perfect pregnancy and ecstatic family anxiously awaiting the birth of this child, he lay in the Georgetown NICU barely alive. There had been no heads-up. One minute Travis was driving us to the hospital while I grasped hold of the dashboard, breathing through contractions; a few days later we were being told to prepare for our firstborn son's funeral. What music would we select? Who would speak? Where do you buy a casket for a newborn? For some, a deep numbness takes over one's body when in crisis and shock; for others, instant shooting pain jabs like knives. We had no idea how this had happened, or how we would survive this excruciating pain. We had been thrown into a journey no one could have ever prepared us for, yet all we knew to do was hold tight to *hope* and each other.

Many people in the world welcome children to this planet we call Earth. Each birth (and life) is important, worthy, and unique, but most births are basically routine: the opposite of extraordinary. Babies are born like clockwork in every city around the world, every minute of every day. The thing about the life of Bennett Mitchell Speck is that very little had felt "routine" from the moment we found out we were expecting him. What looked like a "normal" first-time parental journey turned into one of the most dramatic soap operas, most riveting live theater, and most jolting roller coaster we could have ever imagined.

While I was a junior in high school, for some peculiar reason, our family dentist removed only one of my four wisdom teeth. He said that my wisdom tooth's roots were twisted, and it had to come out instantly during one visit. At the time, all I remember is that he yanked it out with local anesthesia and told me not to eat for an hour. Before I knew it, I was munching on some Pizza Hut pizza at their all-you-can-eat buffet before driving back to high school for my afternoon classes.

A decade later, when I was an established professional, with dental insurance, I got a referral to have my other three wisdom teeth taken out in early January 2007. Leading up to this we had made the decision that we were ready to start a family, but after months of "trying" we thought we were headed toward a fertility consultation. On the morning of my wisdom-teeth extractions, I numbly took a pregnancy test as an act of precaution, per the pre-surgical guidelines. That was their policy, and I had not even thought twice about it. No part of me thought I could be pregnant. I had been extremely irregular with my cycles for years and had several friends who had walked the infertility path. I was fully prepared, and basically assumed that we would be the next couple to struggle to start a family. You can imagine my surprise when a bright vertical line appeared on that little white stick, indicating "pregnant."

I walked out of the bathroom in a stunned stupor as Travis was tying his shoes, getting ready to drive me for the tooth extraction. I slowly placed the pregnancy test on the counter next to him and said, "Look." His eyes peered over to the stick, then he looked at me and said, "Does that mean you are pregnant?" To which I then replied, "I think so!" We looked at each other wide-eyed, hugged, and shook our heads feeling bewildered by this welcome surprise. I called my oral surgeon, told them the circumstances, and they said we would have to cancel; they could not give me anesthesia while I was pregnant. The cancellation of my wisdom-teeth extraction made our reality even more jarring as I had begun to process our pregnancy news. In the haze of a figurative fog, we each got ready for work due to the change of plans and headed into our offices. We told our bosses that "Something had come up and the surgery was canceled." Of course, that small "thing" was the fact that we were having a baby and our hearts were filled with thanksgiving, shock, and joy.

Our pregnancy journey with Bennett included nearly twenty weeks of nausea, some vomiting (at night), constant cravings for carbs to keep my stomach settled, and regular obstetrician (OB) appointments with a highly recommended local practice. I worked full-time for a financial services firm, sitting at a desk all day posting journal entries, updating spreadsheets, and generating financial statements in the cyclical ways that accountants know all too well. The small firm that I worked for was like a family. By my third trimester, the founding partner, a compassionate man and leader, offered me his front-row parking space in the parking garage, and my team laughed at my daily fast-food pregnancy cravings. I was planning to have our baby, enjoy snuggling with him during my maternity leave, and come back to this job that I loved—preferably after hiring the perfect nanny to watch him (a.k.a., a Mary Poppins twin who would love him, sing to him, nurture him, and maybe even teach him a new language). I had even heard of some great nanny-share options near us, so I was confident that our little bundle would be cared for devotedly while we both continued pursuing the careers that we had worked quite hard to establish.

At that time, in the area where we lived, a common sequence of events included spending years getting college-educated, landing internships for "real-world experience," going on to graduate school, law school, or business school, and then landing a solid first job to use as a springboard to propel one's career and pay off the student loans. After one's career was established, the expectation was to work hard to save money for the first house, get married at some point along the process, have children, find top-notch childcare to continue pursuing professional goals, and follow the dreams for your family, however they looked for each family unit. We were subconsciously following this mold amidst the hustle and bustle of the young professional life in Washington, D.C.

When we were in our mid-twenties, Travis and I would probably have been described as low-risk Type-A planners—not super rigid, but we had a "plan." We tried to save money by living in small efficiencies and apartments, we did not travel a lot, and we spent most of our free time with family and church friends. Quite frankly, an outsider looking at us would think we led quite a boring life. We did not have a thriving night life, yet we had a solid circle of friends thanks to our faith community. We each were raised in families of five with married parents and two siblings, and we had a shared value that family was extremely important, but a foundation of faith was most important.

When it came time to find out the sex of the baby at the twenty-week ultrasound, we could hardly wait. The day was circled and highlighted in my paper calendar. I dreamed about that day and anxiously awaited the arrival of the ultrasound appointment that sunny day in April 2007. Because this was my first pregnancy, I did not have a strong feeling about whether we were having a boy or a girl. I knew that my hair was thicker, my wardrobe no longer fit, and I brought crackers everywhere I went to keep my nausea waves under control.

When Travis and I were called into the small room with the sonogram technician, we sat there in complete silence and awe as he waved the wand over my belly. Immediately the black-and-white images of our baby popped up on the small screen. The technician pointed out the baby's head, the belly, the arms, and the legs, checking each inch of the baby's anatomy while making notes along the way. It felt as if the minutes were dripping by like molasses, but finally he asked, "Do you want to know the sex of your child?" and we immediately replied, "Yes!"

Several friends had made the decision to wait until the baby's birth to be surprised at the sex, but Travis and I had agreed that we wanted to know as soon as we could find out. "It's a boy. You are having a boy. Here, I'll show you how I know." A son. Our firstborn child was going to be a son. Travis's family name would continue into future generations, and I would officially be a *boy mom*. I had two brothers myself. My youngest brother, Bobby, was nearly twelve years younger than I, and I had always felt like a second mother to him. I loved boys. We were ecstatic and it all felt almost too good to be true. After the ultrasound, we spent that early April afternoon walking through a neighborhood known for its incredible renowned blossoming cherry trees. As the wind blew delicate light-pink petals through the air, we were filled with happiness as we watched the air fill with light pink "snow," holding hands and processing the joy that our first child was a son.

Once I was well into my second trimester, I left work early once a week to attend pre-natal yoga at a super-hip yoga studio within walking distance of our home. I squeezed into any comfortable workout clothes I could still fit into, walked down the sidewalk of our idyllic tree-lined street, and arrived at the yoga studio to immediately plop on the floor with all the other expectant mothers. While we stretched and "centered" ourselves to New Age yoga music, I glanced around at the other expectant mothers, nervously wondering which of us would be the first to deliver our babies. Some of the mothers looked so confident and experienced, I figured that this was surely not their first baby. They exuded such expertise, like proud peacocks. Some moms looked peaceful and in harmony with the universe, like white swans, while other moms were so very nine-plus months pregnant that I was afraid they might go into labor any moment. Each time I went to prenatal yoga, I was the bloated bug-eyed first-time expectant mom attempting to be chill, centered, and calm, when in reality I was like a nervous, swollen cowgirl trembling in my boots.

During this pregnancy I ate as healthily as I could, I walked regularly, I took my prenatal vitamins religiously, and soaked up my growing baby bump and increasing curves. My hair was truly thicker than it had ever been, thanks to those vitamins packed with nutrients, and I kept pinching myself, reminding myself I was pregnant with our first son. Being a mother was the one consistent dream I had ever had, and yet our families had probably wondered when we were ever going to begin starting a family. Announcing our pregnancy to each of our families was memorable, and the months following included baby showers, gifts, and an abundance of love and support coming our way.

Toward the end of my pregnancy, I even kept a journal in which I wrote to my son growing inside my belly. I hoped that one day he would read these words and see how my love for him was strong, long before he even entered the world. I did not know what my son would look like, what his interests would be, or what he would grow up to be, but I knew that I loved him with every fiber of my being. With each strong kick I felt inside me, I knew that he was destined for great things. I was convinced he would be a world-changer, and I could not wait to watch how that would unfold. The one thing I knew with absolute clarity was that I would love him unconditionally, every minute of every day of his life. Hope was abundant.

CHAPTER 1

Bennett's Birth

ON AUGUST 19, 2007, I woke up to the hot and swampy humidity of a D.C. summer morning not feeling well, immediately feeling "off." I was very tired and achy, but I had read that these symptoms were very possible when a woman is about to go into labor. As a result, I spent most of the day resting and trying to stay cool inside our "little blue house with the red door" rental just steps from the Chevy Chase D.C./Maryland border. I did not dare step outside to be pummeled by the oppressive heat, so I lay around the house all day in front of box fans, trying to stay cool. To be completely honest, I knew deep in my gut that something did not seem normal. I had never felt this way, but I had also never been pregnant before. I took deep breaths, closed my eyes, and tried to relax. If I were about to go to into labor, I wanted to have as much rest as possible.

That evening Travis suggested that we eat dinner at a local favorite D.C. Tex-Mex restaurant, in an effort to cheer me up and get me out of the house—chips, salsa and queso were always a hit (he knew how to motivate me!). I agreed, threw on some clothes over my swollen, large, thirty-eight-weeks pregnant body and waddled to the restaurant for a pleasant dinner. I recall trying to enjoy the good food, spirited music, and upbeat atmosphere with my dear husband, but as we left and headed to our car after dinner I felt especially "off." I even remember standing at the corner of Wisconsin Avenue, staring at the post-dusk outline of the magnificent National Cathedral, one of our favorite sites in D.C., considering going straight to the hospital that minute to see if I was in labor. I stood there contemplating whether I was being dramatic, or if something was truly not right. I knew I was not having any contractions and had read many women's birth stories telling tales of "false alarms," so I concluded the emergency-room doctor would just tell me it was a "false alarm" and send me home. Thus I shrugged it off, slowly ducked into our car, and we headed back to our little blue house on that hot, sticky night of August 19, 2007. Travis fell asleep quickly in our bed while I showered and tried to get comfortable on our futon in the living room. I continued to feel less and less normal, so something within me gently nudged me to check my temperature. I had to dig through our first-aid kit to find the thermometer, as I could not remember the last time either of us had checked our temperatures. And to my fear, the thermometer read that I had a fever of 100.2 degrees Fahrenheit.

As I watched Travis sleep soundly and peacefully, I immediately Googled "fever when pregnant" and called my doctor. Both the Internet and the on-call doctor for my OB practice calmed my worries. The OB advised me to take Tylenol, wait an hour to see if the fever went down, and to call him back in an hour. The fever did go down, so I called him back and he said to call him back if the fever went back over 101. I was able to cling to his calm voice that had been affirmed by those "Internet experts" on WebMD. *Surely this is no big deal. No need to worry. This is all so routine. Doctors see this all the time.*

But that night, lying there "counting the baby's kicks" and reading my Bible, I was anything but calm and free from worry. I was feeling fewer kicks than normal, yet the Internet had told me this was very normal when the baby was full-term and labor was near. As a result, I kept breathing deeply, re-positioning myself, and tried to focus on the daily scriptures for the day. That day's daily readings were from Esther, one of my favorite Bible stories, of a Jewish female leader who rescued her people from oppression and death. Esther chose bravery and I was strengthened by this as I sensed that our upcoming birth was going to require more bravery than I could comprehend.

In a very distracted and unsettled way I got through my daily Bible readings, prayed continuously while trying to get comfortable enough to sleep, and then about 1:30 a.m., much to my surprise, I felt a gush of water come pouring out. I knew that I had not just wet my pants—much to the contrary, my water had just broken. Amniotic fluid came flowing out all over me, the futon, and the Pottery Barn rug beneath me. I was stunned, flabbergasted, excited, soaked, and terrified.

I grabbed my phone immediately and once again, less than five hours later, I frantically called my OB. The same on-call doctor advised me to come right to the hospital. I asked him if I could shower first and he said yes, "but be quick." Immediately I woke Travis up from a deep sleep to give him the unexpected news. I quickly showered, grabbed my hospital bag (already packed), and we were out the door. The painful contractions were happening every three to five minutes in the car as we made our way to the hospital. I breathed through them while slowly counting 10-9-8-7-6-5-4-3-2-1, as we had learned in our hospital class for new parents. As clueless first-time parents, we had been told this hospital was "the place" to have a baby if living in Northwest Washington, D.C. Word on the street was that mothers were treated wonderfully, massages were included after birth, and you could even pay for your own private room once the baby was born. After seven years of marriage and nearly ten years together as a couple, the moment had finally arrived to meet this precious son we had been anxiously waiting for.

Travis dropped me off at the entrance to the emergency room as he went to park the car. Each contraction was getting stronger. I had a towel between my legs as I waddled to the door and could barely finish a sentence. We had pre-registered with the hospital weeks before, so I told the first person I could find that I was most certainly in labor. The triage nurse saw my disheveled appearance, plopped me into a wheelchair, and pushed me right up to the Labor and Delivery floor. As we wheeled into the unit, I blurted to another nurse, "My water broke at home!" She looked at me with a non-amused glance. "Are you sure?" I was taken aback, assuming she had experienced many false alarms in her career, but this was no false alarm! I responded, "Considering my entire futon and rug are soaking wet, and it doesn't smell like urine, I am pretty sure my water has broken. Check me, please!" They quickly realized they now had a feisty first-time mother setting up camp in their ward. Lord help them.

We got settled into our room, the contractions continued to get stronger as the night went on, and eventually I got an epidural (which for a first-time mom was terrifying—to lean forward, hug a pillow, and try not to move during each contraction, all while a large needle was being placed directly into my spinal fluid). Nevertheless, the epidural got placed and things were relatively calm and quiet in our hospital room by about 5 a.m. The nurses told us to try and get some rest while my body had the contractions and my cervix was dilating. They hoped I would be fully dilated by later that morning, in hopes of pushing out our son by that afternoon. It all sounded like a great plan, and we were at peace as we tried to close our weary eyes and attempt to get our last chance at rest for the unforeseeable future.

I do recall quite vividly that I was in a *lot* of pain as the catheter was placed. Nurses were kind and attentive through the night, and I was re-positioned a few times when the baby "didn't look happy," which meant that Bennett's heart rate had dipped per the fetal monitoring system. Yet in the wee hours of the morning, right around the time of the shift change for the nurses and doctors, a new female doctor from our OB practice popped into our room around 7 a.m. to discuss the possibility of a C-section. When she first entered our room we listened and nodded with groggy eyes, but at the mention of an emergency C-section, we were both jolted to alertness. After checking me, the doctor reported that I was not close to being fully dilated and they were seeing continued signs of the baby's possible distress: With each contraction I had, his heart rate went up. The increased heart rate could be a sign of infection, and a C-section was looking more and more necessary.

Although we had previously (and eagerly) attended our "natural" birthing classes there at the hospital, we were honestly completely fine with the C-section option. I was not upset in the least—my own mother had had three C-sections, Travis's mom had had C-sections, and all we truly wanted was a healthy baby. As a result, we decided to trust the doctor's expertise, signed the waiver papers for the surgery, and quickly prepared for an emergency (i.e., not planned) C-section to meet our precious son early on the morning of August 20, 2007.

Within twenty minutes, the doctor was scrubbed up, the operating room was sterilized, nurses gathered, I was wheeled in, and Travis walked in to be seated at my head while a fabric curtain was placed at my chest to block the surgery happening on my abdomen. We were filled with excitement, and I even remember wishing that we had brought in some music to have in the background of this significant moment of celebration and thanksgiving. I had read that idea from mommy bloggers during that time and wished I had planned ahead for just the right playlist. Oh well. We had been waiting in such eager anticipation for the birth of our first child, and finally the thrilling moment had come. Who cares if the background music is not setting the mood as I had envisioned it?

The C-section began while I lay on the cold operating table, shivering quite noticeably due to the anesthesia. Travis has always had an interest in the medical field, so he stared over the curtain to see the surgery taking place, in hopes of catching the first glance of his son. He desperately wanted to see what was going on, so he reported back to me that everything was clicking like clockwork. I lay there, feeling tugs here and there, feeling like I was living in a dream. I could not believe this moment was happening.

Throughout my life I had seen Hollywood-scripted birth scenes in movies and TV shows and had played with baby dolls well past the age of twelve, but now in a few brief moments I was going to get to hold my very own baby. As I felt the final big tug of our son being pulled from my body, Bennett Mitchell Speck entered the world at 9:20 a.m. weighing seven pounds, six ounces and measuring 19 1/2 inches long. Unbeknownst to us at the time, he was born blue and barely breathing. We did notice that he came out not crying as the room was instantly eerily quiet when the medical team pulled him out of me. We later learned that he was barely alive, registering very low Apgar scores, a measure of the physical condition of all newborn infants.

Immediately it felt as though all the air had been sucked from the room, the energy was tense, and we were unsure of what exactly was going on. The nurses quickly cleaned Bennett off, wrapped him up into a blanket, and a kind nurse nervously blurted out, "Here's your son!" as she held him up for us to see his face before running him down the hall to the NICU. We were completely stunned, so all we could do was watch the operating room's door swing back and forth behind her, listening to its dull squeak. Our "birth plan" did not include this. *What on earth is going on?* We had planned to have our newborn son placed on my bare chest for "skin to skin" and his first attempt at breast feeding. Instead, we were left with a silent, cold, and tense operating room filled with medical professionals who seemed to be as dumbfounded as we, the two first-time parents, were.

The moments following Bennett being whisked away to the NICU were the kickoff of a nightmare journey we never could have prepared for. Our hearts were prepared for a healthy birth based on all the indicators leading up to that day, and yet instead of a healthy birth we were experiencing a traumatic birth with a baby in serious life-threatening distress, just moments away from being born stillborn.

SHOCK /shäk/: a disturbance in the equilibrium or permanence of something

Very little was communicated to Travis and me while we were in the operating room. The doctor quickly mumbled that Bennett was being taken to the NICU to have his vitals taken and to be checked out by the NICU doctor. We heard words like *possible meconium aspiration* as I was wheeled into a recovery room, leaving the air in the operating room as thick as a summer night's air over a delta swamp. Travis followed my stretcher in a stupor, and soon thereafter two NICU doctors came in to report to us that our baby's lungs were full of pneumonia. Bennett was having difficulty breathing, and he appeared to be septic (infection was invading his entire body). Due to the level of this hospital's NICU, Bennett was rapidly needing more support than they were able to provide to him. We were told at this point every minute was critical, and there was no time to waste. Travis walked to the NICU to see Bennett and speak to the neonatologist regarding what exactly was going on. After their conversation Travis quickly realized the seriousness of the situation and plans were made for the next steps.

The NICU team quickly asked us to sign papers to have Bennett transported to Medstar Georgetown University hospital for their Level IV NICU. The doctors were recommending "whole body cooling" and Georgetown was able to provide this. Whole body cooling uses a water-filled cooling mattress to reduce an infant's body temperature and treat brain injury that can occur around the time of birth. Georgetown's NICU was the first in the region to offer whole body cooling for hypoxic-ischemic encephalopathy (HIE). For optimal results, this treatment had to be initiated within the first six hours of life. We barely understood what was going on, but we numbly signed the release papers.

To begin treatment as early as possible, the Georgetown NICU team was ready to rapidly transport Bennett to their NICU, three miles from where we were, and a transport team was prepared to come get him. We were completely dazed as Travis sat in a chair next to me and I lay in the bed of the recovery room. It felt as if we had entered the twilight zone, a place where time has no meaning, and yet every moment was instantly critical. It felt as if the world was spinning around us, and I could not see straight or gather my thoughts amidst an array of post-op medications. Forcing ourselves back to reality, we realized it was a foregone conclusion that we had to hand our baby over to these medical professionals. In our minds we had no choice but to trust the medical experts' recommendations while begging God to protect our baby while he was ripped from our arms so unexpectedly.

After signing the release papers for Bennett to change NICUs, the Georgetown Hospital transport team arrived to take him to Georgetown. Within minutes, we were told the transport team was going to leave, but the current NICU medical team wanted us to be able to see Bennett before he left us. We later realized that the team wanted us to have a memory of seeing him alive, if, God forbid, something happened to him *en route* or before we were able to get to him into the new NICU. Travis and I quickly decided that Travis would follow the ambulance to Georgetown while I tried to recover from the emergency C-section and get transferred ASAP. I had been told I was not allowed to be discharged until I could stand up and walk.

Considering I was completely numb from the waist down, I was far from standing or walking.

Travis and I soon noticed in the hall, outside our recovery room, a large plastic box on top of a stretcher. The best way to describe what I saw from my recovery bed was a clear plastic coffin propped up on wheels. The plastic box held lots of cords and machines hooked up to our newborn son, lying completely still inside the box. I could not see Bennett's face—I only saw the size of his unbearably small body. This tiny fella, whom I had barely gotten a chance to meet but loved deeply while he had lived inside me for nine-plus months, was being pulled away from me. As I mustered the strength to wave goodbye to Bennett and the medical transport team, my mind could barely make sense of this unnatural disruption.

Meanwhile, Travis dashed out to his car in the hospital parking garage, jumped into his black 1995 Toyota Camry, and chased behind the ambulance those three miles, jolting him into a new reality. In a flash he had gone from an expectant father to the father of his firstborn son. As a result, he instantly felt a protective instinct mixed with a vulnerability that was inexplainable. Travis later shared, after taking time to reflect on this traumatic event, that as he followed that ambulance with its loud and blaring siren ringing in his ears, he knew that *his life would never be the same.* A short drive that took less than ten minutes did in fact change our lives, our reality, and our perspective for every day following August 20, 2007.

The ambulance went straight to the emergency entrance to get Bennett immediately admitted to the NICU so that the whole body cooling could begin. Travis had never previously been to this hospital wedged in the middle of one of the most historic areas in our nation's capital, so finding the right parking garage to give him the quickest access to the NICU was hurdle number one. After Travis finally found a parking spot, the compassionate concierge pointed him toward the correct set of elevators to get to the NICU. Travis cautiously walked over and entered an open elevator, pushed the button for level three, and after a few brief moments, the elevator doors opened into the third floor. Travis looked left, saw the glass doors with "NICU" clearly displayed, and stepped into the sacred space that would soon become our second home. He told the receptionist that his son had just been transported there. He was asked to sit down in the waiting room, and the waiting began. All around the waiting room were large wooden frames full of pictures of babies who had spent time in the Georgetown NICU. These beautiful children had spent time in the NICU, gotten better, were discharged home, and had grown into strong and healthy babies and children. The NICU staff placed these pictures on their walls in hopes that waiting loved ones would see these NICU graduates and be encouraged. The heartsick family members had no choice but to stare at the precious faces and hope for the same result.

On that muggy day in late August, Travis collapsed into a small chair in the waiting room in a complete state of shock. He was alone, he was weary, and he was afraid. He would eventually look up at those framed pictures lining the walls, grasping for hope as he tried to envision our son following the same victorious trajectory as each of the little faces on the wall. Was there hope?

CHAPTER 2
Get Me to My Baby

"And she loved a little boy very much,
even more than she loved herself."
— Shel Silverstein

AFTER BENNETT WAS BORN, transported to the new NICU, and Travis was with him, I was left stunned and stuck. My devoted mother, Kathy, arrived at the hospital right before the emergency C-section. My mom was there for the NICU team's recommendation to transport him and was there to wave goodbye to her first grandchild, lying in what looked like a plastic coffin. Her grief for the pain she was experiencing, plus watching her firstborn daughter suffer, was almost too much to bear. I saw her almost shaking with fear, but she is a woman of deep faith, had been through a lot in her life, and I could see in her eyes that she was trying to make sense of what was happening. My mother has always been my rock, steady and strong, and she immediately became my advocate—which I needed.

I eventually got moved to a private room, napped on and off, and by that evening was running a fever, was in excruciating pain from the catheter, yet was trying to wean myself from the epidural so that I could stand up and walk. I was desperate to be discharged so that I could be reunited with my newborn son. The first night recovering from the C-section included fever, soaking sweats, and basically torture to my heart. My mom was angry at the doctors and wanted answers; I was in deep shock and anguish at what had happened, and yet in such a fog that I do not even remember talking to Travis for updates that first night. There was no way to make sense of what had happened at the birth, and there was not a thing I could do as I lay in the dark hospital room, watching the moon shine through the blinds on the window. No answers were coming to us other than the fact that I had some sort of infection, was being given antibiotics, and it was time to start pumping because my milk supply would soon be coming in.

What should have been a joyous day following the birth of our son had morphed into a suspenseful nightmare. Smashed were my dreams of welcoming our family and friends into my private hospital room, sitting in my soft fuzzy blue robe, passing around our precious son while sharing his birth weight, length, and birth story over and over, with a smile on my face and the smell of newborn-baby lotion filling the room. Instead, I was watching doctors come in and out with panic on their faces, their lips sealed, and my irate mom ready to blast every nurse or doctor who came in and was incapable of giving her an explanation for this unexpected crisis. What and how did this all even happen?

Bennett's birth in August 2007 was long before social media. I did not even text at that point, plus I had not had a chance to send out an email to let friends and family know what was happening. I later found out that Travis had sent out an email announcing that Bennett was born but was in critical condition, so I was caught off guard when three people from my firm's leadership team, including the founder, came to visit me the day after Bennett's birth. Our firm was very family-oriented and they wanted to be the first ones to welcome the newest member of the team. I recall being embarrassed that I had no explanation for what had happened to our son. I looked horrible after sweating buckets all night (I felt even worse), and was heartbroken that my baby was dying three miles down the road. My kind co-workers popped their heads into my room—their forced smiles and looks of sincere concern will always stay with me. I felt I was watching this all happen from outside and above my body, looking down watching a horror movie, and none of it made any sense. I did not even have tears to cry with at that moment. I was in shock with a dose of denial, desperate to make sense of the tornado sweeping us away.

The next day, August 21, 2007, I was determined to get to my baby. My fever had finally broken and the nurse came in my room that morning to tell me, "Today is the day! You are going to get up and walk today, honey." My epidural had been pulled, the pain meds were now PRN (as needed), and all I had to do was get up and walk to the bathroom a few feet from my bed. *Come on, Kelly. You can do this.*

As Bennett's C-section had been my first-ever surgery, I was not prepared for the pain when standing up for the first time after one's abdomen has been cut open and stitched back up. I will never forget the sensation of being split in two while standing up (bent over) and shuffling ever so gingerly to the bathroom. Yet soon after my first "walk," the nurse checked out my incision, confirmed my urine output and that my gastrointestinal tract was functioning, and said I was cleared to be transported via ambulance to Georgetown that afternoon. My heart could have burst with joy. I was also pleasantly surprised to find out I would be recovering for two more days in Georgetown's labor and delivery ward. *Thank God. I will be in the same hospital as my baby. Get me to my baby. Please, Lord.*

After a few hours of lying in my hospital room begging God to wake me up from this bad dream, the ambulance transport team arrived. Travis was spending every waking moment in the NICU at Bennett's side, my mom had gone ahead of me to Georgetown, and

I was alone with my thoughts. The hospital was eerily quiet as I was wheeled out of my room and down the hall to the elevator, my sensory system taking in every squeak of the stretcher's metal wheels. I recall thinking, "Where is everyone? Why do I still not know what happened to my baby? Did I do something wrong?" Yet there were no answers at this point—only deafening silence as I grimaced with each movement felt by my tender incisions.

The transport drivers got my stretcher secured and locked into the ambulance, and asked me if I was okay. I nodded to them, gritted my teeth, and closed my eyes as I heard the engine turn on. I braced myself, and yet I felt every single bump and curve of the pothole-ridden streets along the journey to my baby and husband. The transport journey was extremely painful both physically and emotionally, and words cannot accurately describe how gutted I felt, both literally and figuratively. Hope was the only thing I had to cling to on that lonely ambulance ride.

CHAPTER 3
ECMO Life Support

"Hope is a waking dream."
— Aristotle

B ENNETT'S CONDITION continued to worsen by the hour. Georgetown NICU doctors were giving him all the medical interventions that they had. He was surrounded by so many machines that you could not even see his newborn body when trying to look at him in his NICU bed. After arriving via transport and settled into my room in the labor and recovery wing at Georgetown, I begged to be taken to the NICU. I did not care that I was swollen, sore, and barely covered in my hospital gown. At this point I had not seen my husband or my son in almost two days, and I needed to be with them. A kind nurse wheeled me down the cold, sterile hall, pushed me into the empty elevator, and the doors opened into the third floor NICU. I was wheeled through the NICU waiting-room glass doors and sat in my wheelchair, staring at all the pictures of the "NICU graduates." My eyes darted around to take in this foreign environment. I watched parents wash their hands in the extra-large stainless-steel sink, and glanced at the coffee area not far away. I saw the worn-out pleather waiting-room chairs lining the congested walls of the waiting room, and the reception desk behind a large glass window across the corridor from the large sink. The room was eerily quiet with an underlying tension that could be felt the very moment my wheelchair was parked.

All NICU parents know that it is one of the most unique experiences in life. Few would ever ask to be in the NICU-parent "club," but once you are in the club, the experiences are etched into your soul. The sights, sounds, and smells never leave you. I was brand new to the club and had no idea how the abrupt initiation into the NICU would present itself. All I knew was that I had been taking my pain meds around the clock and was still wobbly on my feet, but if my baby, whom I had seen only for a brief second in the operating room, was just through the large wooden door, I was determined to see him. I did not know what the protocol was, but Travis soon came out of the secure area of the NICU (behind a large solid wooden door) and we embraced. There was a crowd of people in the waiting room—friends and family—the faces are a blur in my mind, but Travis's strong arms instantly brought peace to my desperate heart. I did not want to hang out in the waiting area—I wanted to see my son—and Travis assured me that now was a good time to come back to see Bennett. My feeble weakness in that moment was instantly given strength by the presence of my tall and strong husband, gently ready to escort me to my son. Travis showed me how to stand at the large stainless-steel sink and wash my hands up to my elbows for two minutes, the strict and standard procedure for all NICU visitors. A kind friend ran over to pull closed the back of my hospital gown as I stood at the sink exposing my bare back and post-birth netted underwear (commonly worn by moms post-partum). I was also asked to put on an additional gown and mask in order to be granted clearance to the secure NICU area. *Clean hands: Check. Gown: Check. Mask: Check. Get me to my son. Please.*

For all the years up to this point I would have considered myself a very non-medical person. I had spent a decade working in sterile corporate America in uninteresting offices filled with tidy spaces and neutral decor. I could not stand to watch my blood being drawn, or even look at the veins on my wrist. But isn't it fascinating how the human body can immediately adapt when in crisis? As I was wheeled into the NICU I did not know what my eyes were about to see, yet immediately an overwhelming peace and deep sense of humanity settled into my heart. I sensed this was our new community of sick babies and hurting parents; these were now our people, and I knew it in the depth of my soul. There were no private rooms in this NICU. The Georgetown University Hospital brick building opened in 1930 and the NICU had not been renovated to provide private rooms for families. The continuous beeping sounds of monitors plus the shared smells of plastic tubing, formula, fresh diapers, and alcohol disinfectants would become our normal sensory inputs. *Dear God, please just give me my baby, and let him live.*

As Travis slowly wheeled me past all the sick babies, I quickly glanced at the parents sitting in gliders next to either isolettes holding premature (preemie) babies, or open NICU bays with high, small beds holding sick full-term babies. By the look of my disheveled appearance, they could probably tell that I was the latest "admitted mom about to see my baby for the first time." I would later see these moms being wheeled into the NICU, and my heart would ache. The parents I was seeing had likely spent days/weeks/months doing this daily routine, yet on that day I was the new member being initiated into their club. I received a few sympathetic smiles, tried not to stare at their babies while we passed them, and finally stopped in front of my son.

The unexpected factor was that unlike all the other babies I had just passed by, I could not see Bennett. His newborn body lay under a light shining down onto his open bay surrounded by machines (a large ventilator), numerous pumps giving him constant medications, plus human bodies of doctors, doctoral fellows, respiratory therapists, and nurses. As Travis gently told them I was here, the bodies parted like the Red Sea, and Travis assisted me up and out of my wheelchair to stand at the side of my precious son. There he lay, completely sedated and still, intubated, full of IV lines going in and out of his body. A week earlier I would have been horrified at this sight, but my eyes had never seen a more beautiful sight. There he was, Bennett Mitchell Speck, the son I had loved with every fiber of my being since the minute I held that positive pregnancy test in my hands. *Hey there, sweet boy. Mommy is here and I will never leave your side.*

Travis and I spent a short time together with Bennett that first evening in the NICU. Bennett was not doing well but was relatively stable, and the NICU doctors were constantly consulting with each other as to the best steps forward. By this point, my mom and dad (both local), Travis's mom Priscilla, Travis's siblings Randy and Meredith, and my brothers Chris and Bobby were flying into town from cities across the country. Unbeknownst to me they had been told there was a high chance that Bennett would not survive his current condition, so they needed to get to D.C. if they wanted to meet him alive. I did not know that they all came for the chance to see him alive, and I am grateful that information was not shared with me; I fear that my newly post-partum heart would not have been able to process such a blunt reality. Logistics were bustling by the hour as my dad picked up family members from the airport and arrangements were made for lodging. Thankfully it was all taken care of without our involvement.

Papers to sign

Because encompassing pneumonia was filling Bennett's lungs, and organs were on the verge of shutting down, Travis came up to my Georgetown hospital room later that first night. He timidly stepped into my room along with a sharp female NICU fellow in scrubs. I immediately noticed that she was holding a piece of paper and I wanted to know what it was for. The fellow said to me, "Hi, Mrs. Speck. Your husband and I came to talk to you about Bennett. We have a decision to make and we need to make it somewhat quickly. Your newborn son is very sick. He is basically drowning. His lungs are filled with pneumonia. We do not believe he will survive." All the techniques tried by the medical team were not working, so the NICU doctors were strongly recommending placing Bennett on a life-saving heart/lung bypass machine for five to seven days to oxygenate his blood for him and give his body some rest. The risks were high: a brain bleed being a top risk, which would require daily brain scans of Bennett's brain to detect any possible bleeds. We were told 80 percent of the babies placed on the bypass machine lived. That percentage initially sounded positive to two terrified and desperate first-time parents. The survival rate has since decreased to 65 percent, per a 2018 study published by the National Center for Biotechnology Information (NCBI).

Travis and I talked quietly for a few moments, going over the pros and cons for doing this procedure. Amidst the fog of my pain meds and Travis's understanding of conversations in the NICU, we each signed the hospital's surgery consent papers. I can still picture in my mind which corner of that hospital room we were standing in, and I recall the way the dim light shone on the paper as our pens danced across the page. The ink from the pens signified that our initials were agreeing to a last-ditch effort to save the life of our son. All we could do in that moment was cling to hope that our son would be part of the 80 percent survival rate.

The fellow briskly snatched away the paper while the ink was still wet, and the surgeon was immediately paged to notify him of the high-risk surgery happening first thing the next morning. Travis and I stayed behind in my room and tried to quickly process what we had just agreed to. We were unable to wrap our brains around the gravity of this decision, so we lassoed our hope onto the 80-percent number. The NICU team bustled around his body, located just around the corner from us, attempting to keep Bennett stable enough to make it through the night as we both attempted to chase sleep amidst the nightmare we were in.

The next day, on August 22, 2007, Bennett was placed on Extracorporeal Membrane Oxygenation (ECMO) therapy. He was three days old. ECMO is a mechanical pump used to provide heart and lung support to critically ill infants. ECMO is a heart/lung bypass life-support system that would be removing his blood from his right carotid artery, running his blood through a machine to oxygenate it, and then pushing his blood back into his carotid artery. Two catheters were placed in his right carotid artery and we were told that once he came off ECMO, he would permanently lose use of his right carotid artery. The procedure to place the catheters went well and we were told, "He is more stable, but still in very critical condition. He has pneumonia, pulmonary hypertension, and his body is septic (full of infection)."

Once the nurses told Travis that Bennett was cleaned up from the ECMO procedure and resting comfortably, Travis came to get me from my hospital room so we could see our son. I had no idea what to expect; I just needed to see my baby. I needed to touch his ten little fingers, stroke his ten perfect toes, and I needed to smell the fragrance of his newborn hair. Travis wheeled me out of my room, down the labor and delivery hall, and through the doors of the NICU. We nervously washed our hands. I grimaced with each movement as my C-section stiches pulled each time I stood, sat, or stretched over the large stainless-steel sink, and I looked to Travis's eyes for a glimmer of reassurance that our baby was going to be okay. He was able to give me a smile, and into the NICU we went to see our son. There is frankly nothing that could ever prepare one to see tubes full of red blood coming out of your newborn son's carotid artery in his neck. It was worse than the worst nightmare I could have ever imagined for my son's life to begin. But this was our reality and we simply had no other choice if we wanted his life to be spared. We kissed his cheeks, we whispered in his ears, and we prayed over him before walking away and letting his body have some quiet time to heal.

I do not recall much about the day that Bennett was placed on ECMO. Perhaps the fog of trauma was just settling in. Perhaps we were relieved that we finally had a concrete plan to stabilize our son instead of optimistically attempting multiple medical interventions and feeling defeated with each negative response. Perhaps we were in the throes of crisis, where pain was setting up camp in the core of our beings but distractions were abundant. Aisha Ahmad, a political science professor who has worked and lived under conditions of war, violent conflict, poverty, and disaster in many places around the world, writes in *The Chronicle of Higher Education* that there are three stages of adapting to a crisis:

Step 1: Seeking out *Security*

Step 2: Opening up to *New Challenge*

Step 3: Embracing the *New Normal*

Step 1: The day Bennett was placed on the ECMO machine we had a sizeable group of family members and friends physically surrounding Travis in the NICU waiting room (and me in my hospital room). The emotional and physical support of these dear people became our *security* in those initial days. Travis and I were not taking phone calls and in August of 2007 we were not even in the habit of texting. Somehow updates were being circulated regarding Bennett's spiraling condition to friends and strangers near and far. Throughout the day, family and friends would appear in the waiting room to come sit with us, never forcing small talk; they were simply willing to be present with us in our pain without saying a word. The presence of our loved ones offered us the security that we were not alone. Our mothers hung out in my hospital room while I attempted to learn to use a breast pump in hopes that my milk would come in to give Bennett nourishment. I had been looking forward to breastfeeding my son for months and now clung to the hope that finally there might be something my body could give to him to hopefully help him.

I began to pump dutifully every three hours around the clock. I had a *new challenge*, and it kept me focused on the mission of helping to save my baby. I felt strong and empowered as I watched my body naturally produce this liquid gold for my son, and yet is one of the loneliest actions a mother partakes of when she sits alone in her bed, connected to a breast pump, longing for her baby. It felt as though my hormones were bubbling up and nearly overflowing, figuratively splashing all over the room walls, as I tried to figure out what I was doing. A woman's body is naturally created to have a milk letdown at the touch of her baby, sometimes even at the sound of the baby's cry. And yet my baby was in a different hospital wing, so there were no newborn smells or gentle coos and cries, only the dull hum and rhythmic pattern of the industrial-grade breast pump pulsating in the still air of my sterile hospital room.

Bennett's first days on ECMO brought some stability, and after three days spent in the labor and delivery wing, going back and forth between my room and visiting Bennett in the NICU, the nurses told me that I had been cleared for discharge. I had been experiencing significant high blood pressure so the doctors were monitoring me, but my blood pressure had stabilized, and the doctors were comfortable with a continued recovery at home. I remember my conflicted feelings sharing my discharge news with family members who were in my room that morning. The sun was shining through my hospital room's windows, smiles and hugs were given, it felt like a small victory to get to go home and be with Travis, and yet I felt empty and sad.

Family members eventually left the room to go see Bennett and Travis in NICU, which gave me some time to get dressed, gather my belongings, and pack up to go home. Hospital discharges always seem to take longer than anticipated, but the nurses helped me along the way, had me sign all the necessary paperwork, and finally my nurse called Travis to ask him to pull the car around to the circle drive.

Within a few moments, I was dressed, nervously sitting alone in my room, and oddly there was not a soul in sight. A medical technician had gone ahead of me with a full load of my belongings on a cart, and yet I recall standing in a cold, cream-tiled hall, holding a vase of flowers sent to me from Travis's beloved aunt and uncle, with not another human to be found. I stood there in the silence as I let the gravity of the moment sink into my soul. I was leaving the hospital after the birth of my firstborn son—without my son. In fact, I did not know if he would ever be coming home with me. I was aware of this deep loss occurring with other parents who left the hospital without their babies, and yet I could hardly fathom that this was my current reality. There had been no forewarning and Bennett was not a preemie: He was a full-term baby who was fighting every second to live. He was the sickest baby in the NICU at that time, so it was time to face a new challenge—going home from the hospital not knowing if my son would ever come home to join me.

As I gingerly walked down the hall, past each of the large solid wooden doors hosting mothers lying in beds behind those doors, I knew that all the staff on this floor knew how grim Bennett's condition was. I assumed the nurses and techs had all gotten busy with other patients at that exact moment, but perhaps their devoted hearts simply could not bear to put on a happy face and wish me all the best. Instead, I was given the opportunity to feel this deep loss on my own in the sterile echo chamber of an empty maternity ward. I was not being wheeled out of the hospital holding my newborn son in my arms, the outcome I had envisioned. Instead I was walking out alone carrying a vase of flowers and some paperwork. I felt the profound loss with each step to the elevator and every jarring moment that passed until I stepped out onto the circle drive. I wanted to scream, weep, and run, but my newly sewn-up C-section body was not able to do any of those things. I was too numb from my pain medication and had too many stitches holding my abdomen together to run one step.

Travis pulled our old black Toyota Camry up the circle drive, and our family members met us there to unload all my belongings from the cart, which had been delivered by the medical technician, into the car. They loaded up our car and not much was spoken as our hearts were too heavy. We gave each other forced smiles and tight hugs with tears in our eyes. Bennett was lying a few floors above us in the red brick building, barely clinging to life, and we were about to get in our car with an empty red and gray brand-new infant car seat. The glaring void was nearly suffocating. The car seat had been a baby shower gift, we had nervously taken it to the local fire station to have them safely install it, and we had daydreamed about what it would be like when our son was safely tucked into the five-strap harness. Now the gray canvas car seat straps lay limp and empty like our hearts.

We would soon drive home to a little blue house with an empty crib filled with freshly washed sheets, an empty changing table stocked with baby booties, baby wipes and new diapers, and an empty wardrobe full of clean baby clothes, all with no baby. The weight of the situation was almost too much to bear, but by the grace of God (and what we refer to as "holy numbness"), we somehow went through the motions. We waved goodbye to our family as we pulled away from the hospital and Travis quietly drove me home. He held my arm as I delicately walked up the three steps to our little house and entered our home without our baby. We attempted to unpack, feed ourselves the food that loved ones had left for us, called the NICU to get the latest status report, and fell into bed hoping we would wake up to find out this had all been one bad dream.

Despite the events of the day, hope was with us. In fact, hope, along with each other, were all we had to hold on to. Our arms were empty and our hearts were shattered; it felt like a fist had just punched through glass leaving edges jagged, exposed, and raw. We should have been experiencing our first night of rocking, feeding, and changing our newborn son, yet instead we were watching our cellphones to see if we would be getting a call to drive back to the NICU quickly to say goodbye.

CHAPTER 4
Thrown Into NICU Life

"Hope deferred makes the heart sick,
but a longing fulfilled is a tree of life."
— Proverbs 13:12

NICU LIFE IS NOT for the faint of heart. Even if your baby spends only a few hours or days there, it is emotionally, mentally, and physically exhausting. I would guess that any parent who has experienced a baby in the NICU would attest to that. Very quickly we realized that we would not be in the NICU for just a few days. The first time I heard a nurse refer to "at least thirty days" I remember feeling as if I had been slapped in the face. Bennett's case was complex and the medical team could not tell us what to expect because they themselves did not know what each day would hold. Due to the many unknowns, Travis continued to work at the federal government. We hoped that once we were able to bring Bennett home, he would then take his paternity sick-leave days he had built up, so at the time it seemed prudent to save as much of his paid leave as we could.

After I was settled in at home, we figured out a new rhythm to adapt to this odd existence that our lives had morphed into. Travis worked all day, and since I could not drive the first few weeks following my C-section, a family member drove me to the NICU to visit Bennett. There were no beds in the NICU, and the nurses recommended that family members rest at home, so this routine was our only choice. I would spend time with Bennett from lunchtime well into the afternoon, and then Travis would meet me at Georgetown for dinner and to spend the evening by Bennett's side. During these quiet evenings we found that it was a good time to get nurse reports, as the hustle and bustle of the NICU usually slowed down at night. This daily schedule immediately became our new "routine" and we quickly adapted to this *new normal*. Our former life was a distant memory. Before Bennett, we were trying to figure out how we wanted to fill our Saturdays, where to eat dinner with friends, and when to exercise, and now we just hoped that our baby's life would be spared. Oh, the irony of life. Hope was our anchor amidst the storms that were rolling in far across the horizon.

If there was an award for "sickest baby in the NICU," Bennett would have won that award hands-down in early September 2007. That said, there were a handful of other very sick babies, and we bonded with their parents immediately, all nervously waiting together in the waiting room day in and day out. We found ourselves instantly bonded with Brady and his parents, Logan and his parents, Peter and his parents, and the parents of a set of boy/girl twins. There was basically no privacy, so we were forced to process daily updates in front of others. We shared each other's victories and wept with each other's defeats. There was one particular moment of defeat that will stay with me forever.

The dad of the twins, like Travis, was tall (probably around 6'5" like Travis) and slim, but he was a brunette while Travis is blond. We had shared small talk while sitting in the uncomfortable waiting room chairs, so we knew that their daughter was very sick with an unidentified condition, but their son seemed to be doing well. The couple's newborn son was actually on the path to being discharged and we were overjoyed for them. One night Travis had come back to the NICU after work, we had eaten dinner together, and were scrubbing up at the sink to enter the NICU. Travis had not seen Bennett yet, so we were anxious to get his most recent update, and hopefully see his eyes open. Just as Travis went to open the big wooden door to enter the NICU, the dad of the twins was walking out of the NICU door toward us. Their eyes met. Travis went to shake his hand and pat him on the back to say hello, but the twins' dad collapsed into Travis's arms. He began to weep and through his sobs he shared that his daughter had just passed away.

I was watching from six feet away, and it felt as if time stood still. Here, in the middle of this atypical place, surrounded by complete strangers, two random fathers embraced with a shared understanding that only a few could relate to. These two men, who stood like tall redwood trees in the forests of California, were crippled with despair and grief. Never in my life have I personally witnessed an example of such humanity shared by two fathers. Travis attempted to console him; I hugged their mother, and we tried to mumble out a few words of encouragement that came to our minds. Yet we quickly were struck by the fact that we were standing on holy ground. It all became jarringly clear. This NICU experience was a juxtaposition of reality where life meets death, smiles meet weeping, and miracles meet devastation. It took a while for us to process the death of this couple's precious daughter. What became crystal clear to us was that nothing really matters when you are left staring at a cold stainless-steel sink, watching the water pouring over your hands, trying to make sense of whether today will be the day that your baby lives or dies.

One afternoon soon after Bennett had been placed on the ECMO machine, I was sitting in the NICU waiting room with my mom.

Bennett was completely sedated while on ECMO (so that he would not move) and the machine was so cumbersome there was really no way for us to sit next to him. We would stand and talk to him, sing in his little ears, and stand to pray over him, but when we needed to sit, we headed back out to the waiting room. My mom and I started off with small talk by the coffee area, but it quickly turned heavy, and the tears began to flow down my cheeks. I blubbered out amidst the sobs, "I knew it all seemed too easy. I got pregnant so easily, the pregnancy was easy, and we were getting to have a firstborn son. Our dreams had come true. But it was all just too good to be true." I had nowhere to run, so I sat in the uncomfortable chair in the public waiting room with tears silently rolling down my cheeks. The reality of our situation was starting to set in, and it was breaking my heart.

During the days and nights that I spent visiting Bennett, I would go to the NICU "Mothers' Pumping Room" where there were three pumps set up in a small room with large vinyl reclining chairs, each behind its own curtain for privacy. It was great to have a private place, and yet the room was the size of a large storage closet. The first time that I nervously entered this dingy room, I recall walking in with all my "pumping" connection tubes and bottle supplies, hooking my breasts up to the machine, and sitting in the quiet loneliness behind my curtain. The tears immediately began to fall. I was weeping for this new reality. Weeping for my baby dying a few rooms away from me. Weeping for the loss of snuggling with my son in our new glider at home, the one that was waiting for him to be rocked to sleep.

As I finished pumping, gathered my belongings, and opened my curtain, I was startled by what was just outside. There, two steps from me, was a beautiful blond first-time mother sound asleep on the small, uncomfortable vinyl couch. The couch was there for mothers to "wait their turn," and her pure exhaustion stunned me. I related to her immediately. She was exhausted. I was exhausted. Her body was depleted as she recovered from her baby's birth. My body was sore and still tender from the recent C-section I was recovering from. She lay there with her designer handbag thrown open, her vulnerability strewn wide open to any stranger who walked in. I too felt completely vulnerable every second of every day as I tried to make sense of what was happening to my son. In my head I wrestled daily with the "what ifs": *What if I had caused his traumatic birth?*, and quite honestly was criticizing myself for ever caring about getting the stupid designer diaper bag that hung waiting for me at my home.

For the four years prior to Bennett's birth, we attended the church that I grew up attending with my family in northern Virginia, in a suburb of Washington, D.C. Travis had actually sung in the worship service the day before Bennett was born. We had a close group of young professionals whom we met with regularly for Bible study, service projects, and community events. Most everyone was living in D.C. far away from family, so in a way we became family to each other. Much to our surprise, on the morning of Saturday, August 25, five days after Bennett's birth, our church coordinated a prayer vigil at the church for Bennett's health and life, and strength for us. The email that went out to the church congregation read: "We encourage everyone that can to come to the building to pray as we lift this sweet family to God in prayer. For those who attend, we will have a sign-up in the worship center for a twenty-four-hour prayer vigil for the Speck family to start on Sunday, August 26. We ask that you pray during your time slot regardless of your location."

On the day of the prayer vigil Bennett was in such a critical state that we did not feel comfortable leaving him, so my mom attended the vigil to represent our family. When my mom got to the hospital later that day, she expressed to us how extremely encouraged she was by the outpouring of support. A few days later, the children's minister sent us a long list of names of friends who had attended the vigil and had committed to lift our family up in prayer. We were extremely touched by these efforts and wished that we could have been there to hug them all. It pained us to not be there in person, but the mere thought of leaving Bennett while in critical condition was unimaginable.

Our friends from our faith community additionally gave us a "prayer pager" that lit up with the phone number of whoever was praying for us in that very moment. Every hour around the clock that pager lit up with phone numbers—most of which we had no idea whose. The "prayer pager" phone number quickly was distributed to friends and strangers all across the country. Their prayers, these simple acts of thoughtfulness, brought indescribable strength to us in our low moments. In the middle of the night, if we were tossing and turning with worry or struggling to sleep, we would eventually hear the low vibration of the pager and see the dim blue light up flash a phone number. In those moments it was as if we were being given a virtual hug and dose of encouragement to press on and not lose heart amidst our grief. Sometimes when we needed a distraction from our pain, we would look up the area codes that we did not recognize, and we were always amazed at the prayer states which were represented. From California to Maine, people were praying on Bennett's behalf for his life to be spared. We were humbled and deeply touched both then and now.

Each day in the NICU was full of "ups and downs." We, along with many others, were told by nurses the old cliché that "It is a marathon, not a sprint." We met incredible doctors, surgeons, nurses, and respiratory therapists, many of whom were at the top in their fields. The warmth of doctors like Dr. A., nurses like Ashley, and traveling respiratory therapist "Big John" gave us reassurance, hope, and comfort as we entered each traumatic day. And yet as Bennett stayed on ECMO, had blood gases drawn around the clock, and lung X-rays taken daily to watch the stubborn pneumonia, little to no good news was being conveyed to us. The demeanor of the team of doctors was consistently measured, cautious, and uncertain, all while trying to remain positive. Regardless, we were clinging to the hope that our baby was going to pull through this! We kept thinking, *Surely, at any moment, the pneumonia in his lungs is going to start responding to the army of antibiotics that are being pumped into his body to fight it. That pneumonia has got to start resolving. How could it not with all the medicines being thrown at it? Seriously, his lung X-rays must start improving. Please, let it be so, Lord!*

While on ECMO, Bennett's body swelled up with excess fluid like a sausage or a marshmallow man. So we needed him to constantly keep peeing to drain all the fluid from his body. We did experience a few moments of comedic escape when one day a huge family battle began over the use of the word "pee" versus "urinate" in terms of a prayer request for Bennett. The doctors had emphasized that Bennett really needed to "pee like crazy." Travis immediately posted this prayer request on Bennett's temporary website that we were using to communicate with family, friends, and supporters, as we knew the prayers would be lifted up for this specific request. When Travis's mom, born and raised in Memphis, Tennessee, read the post, she was appalled that he had used the term "pee" and not "urinate." The family debate heated up, and eventually Travis caved to his mom's request and the prayer plea for urination was revised. Prayers were answered as Bennett did indeed start urinating consistently.

Regrettably, with each passing day on ECMO, Bennett got worse, not better. He was pushed to the highest levels of the ECMO machine; he even went through an entire ECMO machine exchange when the first machine had too many blood clots inside it, which goes without saying is very risky. We stood amazed as we watched the nurses take a flashlight and shine it into the ECMO machine that was oxygenating his blood, searching for blood clots. I recall thinking, "That's bizarre and seems very manual. What if they miss a blood clot with that flashlight?"

Bennett's chest X-rays and blood gases continued to give us bad news, not good news. The more we prayed, and the more the folks around the world prayed (per our prayer pager), the worse the trajectory was looking for Bennett's outcome. The NICU doctors, nurses, and respiratory therapists all knew about Bennett's website, and some would even read our daily updates and all the comments that people from around the country (and world) were leaving. On September 1, thirteen days into the NICU stay, our doctor asked our community of prayer warriors to focus on four specific prayers. First, pray for his lungs to open up and begin the process of working on their own. Secondly, pray for the infection and fluid in his lungs to be reduced significantly. Thirdly, pray for his oxygen levels to increase. And lastly, pray that his bleeding is held at bay. We were all desperate for the trajectory of his case to take some strides in a positive direction.

We began brainstorming with the medical team what else we could do to attack the pneumonia in his lungs. In a desperate attempt to drain the horrible jelly-like fluid lodged in his lungs, we agreed to have a surgeon place two chest tubes in his lungs. Their purpose was to attempt to drain a portion of the pneumonia to free his lungs of this jelly-like bacteria that was holding him, and all of us, hostage. We knew that it was a risky procedure, but his prognosis was getting grimmer by the day, and he could not stay on ECMO indefinitely. We needed his lungs to clear up, and we needed it to happen quickly.

Much to our dismay, the chest tubes simply did not work. The pneumonia was too thick, too stubborn, and refused to drain out of the chest tubes. In the days following their insertion, we were devastated as we watched each chest X-ray come back unchanged. His lungs were still full of pneumonia. Here and there we might see an X-ray that showed a brief improvement, but the next film would show that his lungs were filled again with pneumonia. The numerous antibiotics that he was on were not able to dissolve the monster bacteria in his lungs. Each report of bad news was like being punched in the stomach continuously. Considering at that time we already had either a dull ache or continuous shooting pains in our stomachs, we were battered, we were weary, and we were depleted.

CHAPTER 5
Stop the Bleeding

"God's grace is painted on the canvas of despair."
— T.D. Jakes

WHAT ULTIMATELY BECAME the worst hurdle for us to conquer was the blood thinner Bennett was on for the ECMO therapy. I first noticed that his neck incision site at his right carotid artery appeared to be pulling open, with blood starting to trickle out. He had so many IVs in his tiny body, even a central line in his chest, so immediately my mama bear instinct knew that this was not good. I did not know much about medicine, but had an ill feeling that we were in trouble. We had his surgeons checking the bleeding incisions around the catheters in his neck regularly and they even added a patch to promote active blood clotting, but the patch didn't work as well as they would have preferred. Blood was oozing down the back of his neck, pooling, and the trauma of the sight struck a match to my mothers' intuition. This was getting bad fast.

We absolutely knew from the beginning the blood thinner was a risk, as we had been told the entire time that the risk of bleeding was high. Our concern had always been a brain bleed, but since his brain scans had all been clear up to this point, a false sense of security had set up camp in our minds. That false sense of security was abruptly halted as the blood thinner began to cause significant bleeding from every open line into his body. The chest tubes, which had just recently been placed to remove the pneumonia, soon acted as rivers of blood flowing out his body.

As a result of the two chest tubes which caused the outpouring of Bennett's blood into buckets on each side of his NICU bay, doctors then ordered nurses to perform blood and platelet transfusions, one after another, around the clock, as deemed necessary. Nothing can prepare a person to walk up to see their baby as he has three large tubes of his blood either going in (ECMO) or out of the chest tubes of his body. We surmised that things were dreadfully trending in the wrong direction at a horribly rapid pace.

On the afternoon of September 5, I was in the NICU visiting Bennett, attempting to ask my daily questions, hoping for one glimmer of good news, but the nurse, Amy, would not look me in the eye. Amy's face told me that she was very nervous and most likely very scared. She was a nurse we had had consistently over the past two weeks, and she had never given off this energy. I knew that Amy was a darned good nurse and that she cared deeply for her patients, especially Bennett. But in that moment, Amy could not look at me. I knew in my heart why. The end was near for my son. I watched her talk on the phone with doctors, reporting the high volume of blood that was pouring out of our baby's body, asking for the next order of blood and platelets. She was doing all that she could to keep Bennett stable and safe, and yet his bed was beginning to look like a bloody crime scene.

Travis arrived at the NICU later that afternoon and he immediately sensed that the energy regarding Bennett had shifted, and things were not good. He could tell that something had changed. I could barely offer words to describe the day. He suggested we get some fresh air. I agreed and we stumbled out to the green turf practice field at

Georgetown University to catch our breath amidst the ongoing suf-focating nightmare. At this point in the NICU experience, my shock and trauma were being bullied by deep grief and "mommy guilt" was boiling up within me.

As we walked together slowly, with the sun beginning to set over the Potomac River, I was barely able to look Travis in the eye but blurted, "I am so sorry that this happened. I must have done some-thing wrong. I am so, so, so, sorry. If you are mad at me, I understand why." All I could say over and over as I wept uncontrollably was, "I am so, so sorry." My tears streamed down and bounced onto the turf, we embraced, and for the first time since August 20, we were fully transparent with the thoughts and fears running through our heads. Travis assured me over and over that no, this was not my fault and no, he was not mad at me. My ears heard from him, "It's not your fault," and I was able to find rest in those words. As tears flowed for both of us, it was one of the most honest moments of our marriage. Travis's loving response in that moment was exactly what I needed, and I consider it one of the greatest gifts he has ever given me. Had he been angry and/or blaming me in that moment, I do not know that I could have recovered or continued to function. We stood there hugging and sobbing until there were no tears left to cry.

We did not know what was about to happen, but we knew that we needed more support, so Travis called up his dad, Steve, in Tennessee, and asked him to come immediately. We needed him. We had never made such a request, and Steve knew in that moment that things were very bad for Bennett. Without asking another question, he made some calls to get on the next flight to Washington, D.C. Travis hung up the phone as the early autumn sun was setting over the Potomac River, the changing fall leaves reflecting off the water. It was time to go back to our son. We were completely drained after our "field moment," so Travis and I weakly joined hands and walked back toward the NICU. Our shared commitment to each other, the love and support we were feeling from those around us, and our foundation of faith, were the only things that would keep us standing for the blows that were about to come.

Back in the NICU, Bennett lay fully sedated in his open bay, as pale as a ghost. His skin was eerily white as he lay on his stark white sheet, dark red blood puddling beneath his neck and under the small of his back, where the top of his diaper met his soft skin. As a non-medical person, it was grueling to watch my baby lie there in his own blood, with my gut whispering to me, *This is bad. This is very bad.* Yet I knew I had no control over anything happening in that NICU. There was not one single thing that I could do, other than pray to God and beg all those whom we knew to pray for a miracle.

Bennett survived the night with continuous blood transfusions, and the next day Travis's dad, Steve, arrived at the NICU. Having Steve's strong arms to hug us and help hold us up, literally and figuratively, was a lifeline that helped sustain us. Steve is an extremely generous person; the NICU staff had grown to love him from his previous visits. He arrived trying to be as positive as he could be. His smiles and Southern drawl were a welcomed breath of fresh air as he got up to speed with us and the doctors. But he had spoken to Travis's uncle, an accomplished heart surgeon in Memphis, and he knew the odds were not with us. The medical team was clearly uneasy with how Bennett's condition was trending, and late that afternoon they had a big meeting to discuss necessary steps to take. Surgery to remove the infection from his lungs was discussed, but the surgeon felt strongly that there were far too many risks for internal bleeding to occur, so that door was closed. When that door was closed, we knew that our only hope was a miracle. We needed Bennett's lungs to start working on their own so that he could come off the ECMO machine. The odds were stacked against us; we braced ourselves that we were nearing the end of his life, and yet still, hope was with us.

CHAPTER 6
The End of ECMO

"Tears are the words the heart can't express."
— Gerard Way

O N THE NIGHT of Thursday, September 6, day sixteen of ECMO, Travis and I were frantically called into a small conference room just outside of the NICU. We requested that Steve, Travis's dad, come in with us, and our request was granted. The room was filled with the NICU Division Head, the attending NICU doctors, fellows, and the nurses we had become the closest to. Several nurses were extremely protective of our son and were undeniably personally invested in the outcome of his case. The air in the room was tense, you could hear a pin drop, and our energy was anxious. The fidgety medical team sat in old wobbly fake-leather chairs with wooden arms and tears all over the seats. They sat there, some with stone-cold faces, some with forced smiles, others staring blankly at the three of us—me in the middle, with my hands grasping both Travis's and his dad's hands. There was no time for small talk, so a strained silence permeated the room.

Finally, the Division Head cleared his throat and told us that it had been determined that Bennett was to be removed from the ECMO therapy machine that night, due to the bleeding that was occurring as a result of the blood thinners. We were told to prepare for the fact that he most likely would not survive this procedure. In their opinion, his lungs were not ready to breathe on their own, even with the highest level of jet ventilator that they had. But removing him from ECMO was simply the only option. The next twenty-four hours were going to be critical. Based on his most recent lung X-ray they did not expect him to survive the next twenty-four hours, but if in fact he did survive the first twelve hours off of ECMO, that was a promising sign.

As we sat in our chairs completely stunned, devastated, and grief-stricken, Travis and I could not gather words to respond. *How could this be the end to our story? How do you begin to plan a funeral for a baby? What songs will I want to hear sung as I weep over my baby's casket? What on earth will I say to people as they line up to offer their condolences?* These thoughts were running through my stunned head until Steve, Travis's dad, said, "Thank you, Doctor. We hear what you are telling us and we trust your expertise. That said, we are people of faith and we are going to pray that this precious child does survive. We are also going to ask a host of saints from around the world to join us in that prayer." The medical team all gave us polite smiles and nods, and then, as quick as a pack of jackrabbits, the nurses, fellows, and doctors jumped up to make plans for the removal of Bennett's body from the ECMO machine after sixteen days of dependence.

There was now an electric buzz in the air in the NICU, as bodies buzzed around Bennett's bay like a swarm of bees. We had been asked by the medical team to stay in the waiting room until the procedure was complete. The ECMO catheter removal surgery was going to take several hours, so they encouraged us to get some food, send out emails, and perhaps even go home quickly to get a change of clothes and toothbrushes as it was going to be a very long night.

Right away we gathered together and prayed harder than I have ever prayed in my entire life. Steve, my mom, Travis, and I huddled together in the conference room, arms wrapped around each other tightly, and we cried out to God in utter raw desperation. I merely remember begging, "Please, Lord! Please, Lord! Please, Lord!" over and over through endless tears as Travis's dad prayed on Bennett's behalf.

Travis immediately went to find the public computer in the parent lounge, a more private family waiting room for parents only—a place to sleep, eat, or be alone out of the public waiting room area. He knew that we needed every person of faith that we knew to start storming the gates of heaven with prayers for a miracle for our son, Bennett Mitchell Speck. We had people from Honduras to Maine, from Texas to Great Britain, lifting up Bennett by name, begging the Lord to spare his life. At that point in 2007 we were not participating in social media, and had not even really started texting yet. Bizarre, we know! But regardless, at that point in time email and a generic website that we updated daily were our main two outlets to communicate Bennett's status updates to our support networks.

It is nearly impossible to eat when you know that your child might or might not be surviving the next twelve hours of life, but we shoved down a few bites in the Georgetown student union food court to then quickly return to the NICU waiting room, our home away from home. It might have been hours, but after what felt like thirty minutes one of our most loved nurses popped her head out and said, "Everything went perfect. Bennett is stable and breathing on his own. The next twenty-four hours are crucial, but we want you to come see him." We quickly scrubbed in, flew through the brown wooden door and made a beeline for our baby. As we walked up, we saw what appeared to be a tiny angel lying on a white cloud.

Gone were the huge machines and the blood pooled around him everywhere we looked. Bennett was completely cleaned up, the catheter tubes removed from his carotid artery, and he was lying in a bed of crisp white linens with the most peaceful smile on his lips. We wanted to pick him up and never let him go, but he was now reliant on a powerful jet ventilator to keep his lungs opened up, so we stood over him, praising God for this miraculous moment. There is a picture of both Travis and I, admiring our precious baby boy as he lay on the white sheets without the dark red tube pulling blood out of his carotid artery. He lay on his bed of white linens like an angel, his skin getting pinker with each passing moment. Bennett had been immediately taken off the blood thinners, the bleeding from every open line had ceased, and now oxygen was able to freely infuse throughout his body. The miraculous sight of our preciously pink infant son simply took our breath away. There is a picture of this exact moment that we have framed in Bennett's bedroom. Travis's sister gave us the most perfect large frame that holds this picture. Inscribed along the bottom of the frame: "Life is not measured by the number of breaths you take, but by the moments that take your breath away."

What we experienced that night we would not wish on our worst enemy. Watching our son nearly bleed to death right before our very eyes—seeing his blood literally gushing out of chest tubes into canisters on the ground; the canisters were collecting the blood flowing out from his blood transfusions—is one of the most traumatic events a parent of a newborn could ever witness. These sights were a trauma embedded in our minds and hearts, and are ones that will never leave us. Through counseling, journaling, and processing it with one another, we have come to a place where we can talk about it objectively—and yet each autumn when the weather changes from the summer's hot humidity to the cold, crisp taste of fall, my body goes back to that night and my mind sees every detail, my nose smells the sterile aromas, while my ears hear every beeping sound of the machines. Shock, trauma, and hope can absolutely co-exist in the same life experience, and in the days following Bennett's birth they were tightly intertwined like the thickest rope.

CHAPTER 7

There is No Medical Explanation

"There are only two ways to live your life. One as though nothing is a miracle. The other is as though everything is a miracle."
— Albert Einstein

ONCE BENNETT HAD been removed from the ECMO machine, there was a tense yet cautiously optimistic energy humming in the NICU. The medical team wanted Bennett to pull through and live, as much as we did, but there was no way they could say anything more than the facts. The medical professionals were not about to sell us false hope. Bennett remained stable on the jet ventilator after midnight, past 1 a.m., and as we approached 2 a.m., the staff encouraged us to go home to try and get some rest for a few hours. The nursing team promised us that they would call us if his condition changed for the worse. The thought of leaving Bennett in the NICU after such an emotional night was very difficult—no part of us wanted to leave him. Yet we could rest in our utmost trust in the nurses caring for him (by this point it had been more than two weeks since he came to Georgetown), and they had earned our confidence, so we decided to go home to sleep in our own bed.

We went home to our little blue house rental, phoned the NICU the minute we walked in the door, and they reported that Bennett was still stable. Based on the risks that the doctors had shared with us earlier that evening, it felt as if Bennett's condition could nosedive at any moment. The stimulation of the past eight hours had us bug-eyed and awake, barely able to process what we had just experienced. And then the wave of physical exhaustion swept over us, and we collapsed into our quilted queen bed to try and give rest to our weary bodies. Immediately when our eyes opened early the next day, we phoned the NICU and received great news: Bennett had remained stable all night long, with no steps backward so far. He was on the highest level of support from the jet ventilator, and thus far the jet ventilator was giving him what he needed to breathe and produce acceptable blood gases. To say we were relieved is a major understatement. Bennett was still alive and that simple fact gave us the strength to face another NICU day.

We quickly showered, grabbed a bite to eat, and ran back to the hospital to be by Bennett's side. At that point we were about sixteen hours post-ECMO removal, and we knew that we had about eight more hours until we were out of the woods. After we were back by Bennett's side we were encouraged. He was holding steady. Bennett's body was not making drastic improvements that first day; in fact, he was requiring the maximum support of the jet ventilator, and we had no alternative option. This was our last resort. He was stable and not tanking, so we attempted to focus on the positive and not ponder the "what ifs" if the jet ventilator was unable to give him the support that he required.

Throughout the NICU stay thus far, Big John, the gentle giant traveling respiratory therapist, was working on Bennett's lungs every three to four hours around the clock. After Bennett had been removed from the ECMO machine, John was even more determined to get those lungs to open up and resolve the pneumonia. We could sense John's frustration that the treatments were not working as quickly as he would have liked for them to work. We understood his frustration but appreciated his efforts and kept asking our prayer warriors around the world to pray for supernatural healing. We chatted with John more and more, learned more about him and his family, and were touched that he seemed genuinely determined to help our son.

Bennett continued to stay stable well past the first twenty-four hours, and we cautiously celebrated with our nursing team that we had survived the first day post-ECMO with measured high-fives. This was a huge victory and we did not want to take his positive response for granted. We continued to ask for our team of prayer warriors to pray that God would bring healing from the pneumonia. We waited, and we waited some more. There was so much waiting, but eventually we went home to sleep during night two of post-ECMO removal. Each moment was like lying in a hammock over a large black hole. We felt safe and carried while he appeared stable, but we did not know which direction we were heading as the hammock rocked: headed to safety or to a free fall.

As we were knee-deep in the fog and alternative universe of NICU life, time still had no real value after Bennett was off ECMO. It very much felt like a hurry-up-and-wait scenario each hour of every day. Everything was jolted the following day, Sunday, September 9, when we arrived at the NICU to hear of a miracle. It was Sunday, the Lord's day, and something about that day felt different. When Travis and I entered the NICU on that Sunday morning, the looks on the faces of our nursing team, NICU doctors, and John the respiratory therapist, were priceless. They looked at us like it was Christmas morning and they were bursting to tell us what our surprise Christmas gift was. We had no idea what was happening.

"We have incredible news to tell you, Travis and Kelly. Early this morning, Bennett's lungs just opened up. They literally just opened up. We have no medical explanation for what has taken place. We took his blood gases first thing this morning and they were not great, so an hour later his blood gases were checked again, and they were nearly perfect. The lung X-ray shows that his lungs have cleared significantly so we have been turning down the settings on the jet ventilator. If he continues to improve like this, we should be able to remove him from the jet ventilator very soon. We have never seen anything like this." *Hope was here.* Hope was rushing through his corner of the NICU in direct contrast to the stale air vacuum of previous days. Yes, we had grown weary and had tried to prepare our hearts if Bennett did not survive. But hope was stubborn, and hope was sticking around. Clearly this story was far from over.

I can still remember the joy in the faces of our medical team that Sunday. The doctors, respiratory therapists, and nurses could not help but smile big when they walked past Travis or myself. The nurses who cared for Bennett that day had an extra pep in their step. There was a renewed sense of mission and focus on getting this baby well. The air in the NICU that day felt lighter, and our hearts were filled with thanksgiving. There was "no medical explanation" for what had happened to our son's lungs. Many people would wonder how two lungs filled with pneumonia at eight in the morning could be significantly improved within a few hours, with nearly every vital sign seemingly spiraling downwards just moments earlier.

Yet we knew what had happened. It was no coincidence. There were many people praying for this baby around the world. There is no way we could quantify the number of people or the number of prayers that had been lifted up on Bennett's behalf. People from all faiths, people with no faith, and anyone in between had been touched by the life of this tiny boy who was fighting for his life in an NICU in Washington, D.C. We had Protestants, Catholics, Mormons, Jews, Muslims, atheists, agnostics, and everyone in between praying for this child. Bennett's life had touched people's hearts and his story had reached across all religions.

Whether it was in the darkness of the night, in the light of the day, in the quietest personal moments, or in the most public stages, Bennett's name had been lifted up with these desperate pleas: *Please save him . . . Please don't let him die . . . Please heal his weary little body . . . Please send your angels to surround him . . . Please show us your power, Lord.*

Travis and I were stunned, overjoyed, and in shock that our son's lungs had just "opened up." We did not fully grasp the enormity of the reality that we were amidst a miracle, but we knew we could not stop smiling. We stayed focused on the moments we had by his side, stroking his fingers and kissing his cheeks, all while trying to break our learned habits of watching the blood oxygenation numbers on his monitor like hawks. On that Sunday morning God decided to rock the halls of the Georgetown NICU by opening up pockets in Bennett's lungs, allowing much better airflow and function. Many prayers were spoken like those above, many in the name of Jesus, and for some reason, and only God knows why, Bennett was pulled from the valley of the shadow of death. God decided to blow us all away. Hope was still alive.

Yea, though I walk through the valley of the shadow of death, I will fear no evil: for thou art with me; thy rod and thy staff, they comfort me. You prepare a table before me in the presence of my enemies. You anoint my head with oil; my cup overflows. Surely your goodness and love will follow me all the days of my life, and I will dwell in the house of the Lord forever. — Psalm 23:4-6

After sixteen days on the ECMO machine, and a successful ECMO removal, Bennett's lungs were finally starting to make significant strides in the right direction. The energy from the NICU team was still cautiously optimistic and measured, but those we encountered appeared quite cognizant that this child had inexplicably beaten a lot of odds. We got congratulatory hugs from other NICU parents in the waiting room who had been with us day in and day out, and sweet nods from "new" families who had just arrived and did not know details of our story. It felt like an unexpected gift for all in the NICU to have him still with us, and much to our surprise we had a few more unexpected gifts to come that week.

The first surprise gift came the day after Bennett's lungs had "opened up." Bennett's carbon dioxide and oxygen levels were making dramatic improvements at record pace, exponentially faster than the slow improvements of the previous twenty days. That Monday morning Travis headed into his office with pep in his step, and upon my arrival at the NICU to see Bennett, Maureen, another favorite nurse, was standing next to Bennett with a beaming smile. I asked her what was going on, assuming I would be hearing good news based on her body language. She excitedly informed me, "Today is the day we are going to turn off the jet ventilator! Bennett's blood gases are telling the team that his lungs are ready. This is a huge step forward." If he responded well to coming off the jet ventilator, he could be moved from the open bay to a closed crib, and hopefully one day soon we could hold him. Maureen has the biggest and bluest eyes, and they sparkled with excitement as she asked me, "Are you ready to push that button?" All I could do was shout a determined, "Yes!" Big John, the respiratory therapist, was standing right there beside me to show me which exact button to push. We all counted down, "Five, four, three, two, one!" and then I took my right hand and turned that high-powered jet ventilator off. We have a photo of this glorious moment which

I cherish deeply. The significance of that "off" button encompassed the most challenging mountain of our lives up to this point. It is one thing to hear stories of near-death experiences or perceived miracles; it is another thing to experience a mountain literally being moved and witness it with your own two eyes.

The second gift came after what had been a somewhat "normal" NICU day for Bennett. Travis had gone to work, we met up for a quick Subway dinner, and then it was time to scrub in at the big stainless-steel sink. As we walked back to Bennett in his crib, one of our very favorite nurses, Ashley, was standing there beaming. She could not contain her excitement and blurted, "Do you know what day it is?" Travis and I looked at each other somewhat bewildered, having no idea what she was talking about. Ashley announced that the day had finally come for us to hold our son. Bennett was more than three weeks old and we had never held him. We knew his scent and the softness of his skin because we had rubbed his face, head, arms, and legs day in and day out; but we had not had the gift of holding his tiny body in our arms. Our hearts longed to cradle him, rub noses up close, and to count each finger with delight. Finally we would experience this most sacred moment.

We turned around to find two rocking chairs set up next to Bennett's crib, and we each took a seat. Bennett was still intubated and had monitors and IV lines all over him, so there were a lot of cords to maneuver as Ashley prepared to hand Bennett over to me. It was slightly nerve-wracking because I did not want to accidentally yank anything out of him, so I remember closing my eyes and taking a deep breath. I opened my eyes to see Ashley gently lifting him up and out of his crib, his sweet face still super swollen from all the aftereffects of ECMO. I extended my arms, pulled my baby toward my body for the first time since he was pulled from my body, and closed my eyes to feel the power of the moment. Travis's dad had flown home to Tennessee but his mother Cilla was now with us, so Travis and Cilla sat in gliders next to me to *ooh and ahh* at Bennett, take pictures, and celebrate the miracle of this moment. Travis was next in line to hold Bennett, and I was overcome with emotion as I watched his two enduring arms cradle his fragile son close to his strong chest for the first time.

After a few moments of holding his son, the child who shares his middle name and would carry on his family's legacy, Travis passed Bennett to his mother. Cilla then held her grandson for the first time while soaking in all her Grana snuggles—"Grana" being the "grandma name" given to her by her oldest grandson, Palmer. One of Grana's most "famous" sayings as she comforted her kids and grandkids through the years was, "Well, bless his bones." There was never a more perfect moment for Grana to whisper, "Well, bless his bones," into the ear of Bennett, this precious child who had beaten the odds and whose name means "Little Blessed One."

These beautiful moments were stored up in our hearts and breathed new life into weary parents and loved ones. After weeks of heartaches and blows amidst relentless prayers, it finally felt as if good news was possible. That changed the following morning. We woke up under the bright skylights in the little blue house, planning to shower and go off to work and the NICU. Yet I woke up to a missed phone call from the NICU, made in the wee hours of the morning. When I saw the missed call, my stomach immediately sank. The missed call had to be bad news. Good news usually came when we got to the NICU and talked to the nurses face to face. I honestly did not want to return the phone call, because I was not prepared to process what they had to tell me. But then it hit me like a ton of bricks that our baby lay in the NICU all alone, the hospital had tried to reach us, and I did not even know if he was alive at that moment.

I braced myself and immediately dialed up the NICU. The receptionist answered, paged Bennett's nurse, and I sat waiting on hold with each second feeling like an eternity. Finally the nurse picked up and immediately reported to me that Bennett had a prolonged heart-rate spike in the night, which suggested to the medical team that he was most likely having seizures. He was still highly sedated due to his intubation, so he was not exhibiting any other particular physical indication. His eyes had not rolled back, nor was his body convulsing. They had ordered an EEG for that day, had started some anti-seizure meds, and would be monitoring him closely. *Punched in the stomach again.*

I immediately wanted to vomit. I had not seen this blow coming. His brain scans had all been good during his days on ECMO, he had successfully been removed from ECMO, the pneumonia in his lungs was improving, he had been removed from the jet ventilator, and we had just been able to hold our baby. How could he now be having seizures? It was more than I was able to absorb. His lungs and body had been our daily focus, and now his brain was of major concern. I got in the shower and wept as the hot water ran down my body. *Why, God, why seizures? Have we not been through enough?*

Soon after hearing about Bennett's possible seizure activity, we asked our prayer warriors around the world to beg God to take away any and all seizures that he may have been experiencing. We did not know exactly what was going on in Bennett's brain (the EEG results were inconclusive), so we began the familiar dance of receiving bad news, praying for a miracle, and waiting to see what God had in store. Bennett remained on the seizure medications while in the NICU, and all we could do during that time was hope it was a fluke and continue cheering our boy on toward his recovery.

Nurse Ashley's thoughts

There are about four or five babies that I have cared for in my nineteen-year nursing career that have left a lasting impression on my heart, and Bennett Speck and his loving family is one of them. He also holds a rank as one of the sickest babies I have ever cared for, and one of the biggest fighters. That is a whole lot of ranking positions at such a young age!

When Bennett arrived at Georgetown University Hospital, we knew he was going to give us a run for our money. We also knew there was something very special about this child and we would do everything in our power to help him get better. During Bennett's time on ECMO, there were many shifts where I held my breath for twelve hours, but there were just as many that opened my eyes to the fact that we were not in control of whether Bennett stayed with us or left in the hands of Jesus. I watched his sweet family pray over him, surround him with love, and give thanks for him no matter the outcome. After many years have passed, I can still see his dad leaning over him and singing to him, like he so often did, as if it just happened. There is no doubt in my mind that the reason Bennett not only survived, but has thrived, is because of his entire family's steadfast faith.

One of the most pivotal days for Bennett was a day that seemed hopeless. His parents and caretakers gathered in a room to discuss the next steps. It seemed as if we were at the end of the line, and we very well may have been, medically speaking. Bennett was losing blood faster than we could replace it. He had been on ECMO almost longer than was safe without potentially causing more harm than good. I'm pretty sure this was a day where we were all working through the tears. But none of us ever gave up, and him making it through one minute turned into him making it through an hour, then a shift, then a day, and, finally into "Bennett made it!" Truly, nothing less than a miracle.

During his time with us in the NICU, I claimed Bennett as "mine." (However, I'm pretty sure several other nurses did as well!) I'll always remember the honor I had of placing this sweet baby boy in his mama's arms for the first time. What a wonderful moment that none of us knew would ever come or not! Another memory etched on my heart is the day we staged turning off the jet ventilator. In all of the excitement, we forgot to take a picture of his mom turning it off! That was okay, though, because *we just pretended to do it a second time and snapped a picture! I have so many other fond memories of caring for this fighter after the initial storm: giving him his first bath, helping him learn to take a bottle; many, many midnight snuggles.*

Aside from the seizure scare, Bennett continued to make strides in his recovery. The swelling of his head and body continued to subside; the residual fluids were from ECMO. Per the encouragement of our nurses, there were certain upcoming milestones getting closer by the minute. Some days it had seemed as if they would never happen. These milestones should include Bennett moving from his NICU bed (bay) to a crib, wearing clothes, and drinking from a bottle. They were such simple and normal experiences for any other baby following its birth, but for us these were never guaranteed. Now that some routine NICU milestones seemed within our grasp, we were filled with an extra measure of hope.

As the cool, crisp air continued to greet us each morning when the door opened to head to the hospital, what seemed to be an ordinary visit to the NICU in late September was not. I walked into the NICU just before lunchtime and was shocked to see that not only had my baby been placed in a crib, but dressed in a blue, fuzzy, footed-pajama outfit. I was blown away. He looked so cozy, warm, and ready to snuggle. My heart leapt at the sight of Bennett lying there. Until that day, he had been in a diaper bare-chested with leads covering his chest, swaddled in blankets, or wearing cotton hospital shirts and socks. He had not been able to wear one single piece of his newly gifted wardrobe, and staring at his clothes hanging lonely in his wardrobe or folded at our house was a daily source of pain and emptiness each morning as I got ready to visit him.

It was an indescribable gift, as a brand-new mom walking into the NICU, to see my baby fully dressed and lying in a crib. I was overcome with joy. Many people might think, "Clothes and a crib, what's the big deal?" These items are so basic, and yet they flooded me with feelings of normalcy: *This actually feels normal for once.* Up to this point in Bennett's life, nothing had felt normal. In fact, later on, the husband of one of my dear friends summed it up perfectly when he said, "Man, you guys really got baptized by fire into parenthood." I could not have said it better myself. There is no way we could have been prepared for the traumatic takeoff to our parenthood journey, and frankly we most likely would have rather not been given a warning that our experience would be so ghastly.

There were a lot of sick babies. On many of the days we were in the NICU it was completely full, with no empty beds or bays available. Over the weeks we got to know a handful of the other parents. One mom in particular was quite memorable. This mom was a local D.C. resident, and her son had been born a micro-preemie, weighing less than two pounds. Her son was slowly growing and gaining weight, yet his NICU experience had highs and lows similar to many of ours. This mom always came to the NICU dressed well, each hair in place, wearing impeccable makeup, with her fingernails and toenails looking really good. At this point in our NICU journey we were more than four weeks in. I was still wearing my maternity clothes, I had not had a haircut, and my fingertips and toes had not had any attention in months.

We were swapping baby updates and enjoying small talk in the NICU waiting room, as we did most days when we saw each other, when she said, "Girl, you need a pedicure!" I looked down at my toes, realized she was 100 percent right, and yet I knew that I would not be mustering up the energy for a pedicure any time soon. I knew this because I woke up each morning with a nauseous pit in my stomach, partnered with a dull ache that lingered all day. The ache would dissipate the minute that I got to Bennett's bedside, but the dull ache would return upon each bad report. I wearily woke up each morning, showered, ate, got dressed, drove myself to the NICU parking garage, and simply had no bandwidth to make a pedicure appointment. In fact, I wondered if I would ever get another pedicure. Would life ever feel normal again? I could not even begin to picture what my new normal would look like. I hoped that my life would involve holding my infant son in a Baby Björn while walking the tree-lined sidewalks of Northwest D.C., but the realist inside me knew that I could be regularly visiting my son's grave at a local cemetery. All I could do was buckle up, hold on tight, and wait to see what was around the next corner.

Following Bennett's birth I was on maternity leave from my job, Travis continued working to save up his sick and vacation days for when Bennett came home, and there were many unknowns as to what the cost of his NICU stay was going to be, what insurance was going to cover, and if we were going to start receiving huge hospital bills at any moment. One afternoon while I was at home waiting for Travis to get home from work so we could head up to the NICU for the evening, I stood by our desk opening up the mail, bracing myself for the first large hospital bill. Instead, I tore open a thick envelope from a Texas post office. I was stunned to see that many of our friends, and some strangers we did not even know, had pulled together a large sum of money on a VISA gift card to help feed us while Bennett was in the NICU. We were shocked and humbled by this outpouring of love. Thanks to such generosity, we were fed for weeks to come. This kind effort, coordinated by a dear college friend, blessed us by meeting our physical need for food, took away a significant expense during a stressful time, and sustained us along our journey.

Our landlord at the time was a father of two young boys and was equally kind to us in the early days following Bennett's birth. He had voiced his support to help us out with "anything we might need" and his wife kindly gave me a "new mom's survival kit." Imagine our surprise when our landlord soon notified us that an anonymous friend or family member had paid our September 2007 rent to alleviate that burden during our time of deep crisis. To this day, we do not know who this saint is, but thank you from the bottoms of our hearts. Your gift will never be forgotten, and we will one day pay it forward when we see a young couple in crisis. These two generous gestures that met our basic needs of food and shelter touched us deeply. These gifts met our physical needs, but these tokens of charity also made us feel less alone in a time of great pain and disillusionment.

The loneliness of NICU life, especially that of a child teetering on the brink of death, is hard to put into words. The daily tasks of taking care of our physical needs, Travis continuing to work to provide for our family, staying emotionally and physically available to Bennett with all his medical decisions/procedures taking place, and communicating with family and friends was more than a full-time job. All the families who walked this journey before and after us, with additional children to care for: We applaud you and salute you. Bennett was our first baby; we did not have to care for any other children along this journey. If we had had other children at that time, I simply do not know how we would have managed it all. Bennett's NICU days sucked every ounce of energy out of us. As a result, there was very little time to connect with others, let alone each other, to tap into the deep sadness, loneliness, and isolation that was welling up within our hearts.

During our NICU journey we had friends and acquaintances reach out to us who had experienced stays in the NICU, along with other friends or family members who were doctors, nurses, or therapists. Each of these kind people took the time to offer words of encouragement, advice, and hope; we honestly held on to every word that they shared. We sincerely appreciated every message sent our way.

Yet amidst all the encouragement from loved ones and veteran

NICU parents, there was an awareness within the depths of my soul that told me we were somewhat walking uncharted paths—paths very few people had traveled. How many other parents had given birth to an almost dead baby, watched him almost bleed to death, watched him swell up with so much fluid that he looked like a marshmallow baby, saw him almost stop breathing on multiple occasions, watched him scream in agony due to what we thought was morphine withdrawal, spend nearly six weeks intubated, teetering on the need for a tracheotomy, and survive it all, with the possibility of seizures now on the table. The sum of all these experiences left us wandering the halls of the hospital like shells of our former selves. Most days we could give ourselves a pep talk to face the next nurse's report, and yet on some days, especially on Sundays, it seemed as though the weight of the unknowns tore over us like a tidal wave. Little did we know the biggest blow was just about to come. Hope was about to meet its biggest challenge face to face. Would it be the victor?

CHAPTER 8

MRI Results

FOR THOSE WHO are familiar with the Bible, the number forty is quite significant for both Jews and Christians. The number forty is mentioned 146 times in Scripture, and the number forty generally symbolizes a time of testing or trial. Two of the best-known examples are the story of Noah and the ark, and the testing of Jesus in the desert. In Genesis 7:12, Scripture tells us that while Noah was on the ark with his family and all the animals, it rained for forty days and forty nights. In Matthew 4:1-11, Scripture tells us that after being baptized by John the Baptist, Jesus was tempted by the devil for forty days and nights in the Judaean desert, spending that entire time fasting. Other well-known Bible stories include Moses spending forty days and nights on Mount Sinai receiving God's laws, and Jonah powerfully warned ancient Nineveh, for forty days, that its destruction would come because of its many sins. We are not superstitious people who pay a lot of attention to certain numbers throughout life, but we could not ignore the fact that day forty turned out to be significant.

On day forty of our hospital stay, the neurologist sat Travis and me down in that same small, stuffy meeting room just outside of the NICU. Bennett's lungs had improved greatly, and the medical team was ready to extubate him (i.e., remove the breathing tube down his throat that was assisting him in breathing). Before doing so, they needed to conduct a routine magnetic resonance imaging (MRI) that they do on all ECMO babies prior to extubation. At the time we were not really all that worried about the MRI; we were grateful that he was alive, and simply asked friends to pray that the procedure would go smoothly so he could immediately get the breathing tube removed from his throat. Removing the breathing tube was a major goal that we were acutely aware of, as it would be one step closer to getting our son home. By removing the breathing tube, we were avoiding a tracheotomy, which had been a top fear of mine thus far in our NICU stay.

Travis and I casually entered the small conference room and non-chalantly sat down in chairs across from a gray-haired, plump neurologist. Also in the room was an NICU neonatologist whom we had come to know quite well. The fidgety neurologist kicked off the meeting with a forced smile but then cut to the chase by bluntly saying, "The MRI of your newborn son shows severe brain damage. He will no doubt have a cerebral palsy diagnosis, most likely with a seizure disorder as well . . . He most likely will never walk, talk, or eat by mouth . . . Our social worker is right here to meet with you as we know this is the most devastating diagnosis that a parent can receive. She will help to answer your questions and find the resources that you will need once you leave the hospital." Seeing the look of pure terror on our faces, the NICU neonatologist we had a relationship with piped in with his strong Indian accent, "What he is trying to tell you is that the MRI has some areas of concern. We do not know the exact prognosis for Bennett, but with early intervention therapies, children's brains have a way of regenerating and are actually quite resilient . . ." The neonatologist was attempting to sugarcoat the cold, hard, honest truth, and we knew it. Bennett had experienced significant brain damage due to oxygen depletion, which would significantly affect his future development.

"Cerebral palsy refers to a group of neurological disorders that appear in infancy and permanently affect body movement and muscle coordination. Cerebral palsy (CP) is caused by damage to or abnormalities inside the developing brain that disrupt the brain's ability to control movement and maintain posture and balance. The term cerebral refers to the brain; palsy refers to the loss or impairment of motor function." (National Institutes of Neurological Disorders and Stroke)

Travis and I sat there in the uncomfortable wooden chairs, gripping the cold vinyl cushions (once again noticing the rips here and there), but honestly, it felt as if the cushions had just been pulled out from beneath us. We had been sucker-punched in every sense of the phrase. We sat there mumbling out a question or two for the doctors, bewildered and dazed, in a stupor. Certain words stuck out more than others as our brains began to try and process the information we had been given. "Left side is more compromised than his right side," and "He may or may not be able to walk; you will need to start doing intensive physical and occupational therapy immediately." Our roller coaster ride had just ramped up, throwing us into free fall down a ten-thousand-foot drop with no slowdown or end in sight.

Instantly we were filled with conflicting feelings and emotions. After numerous unexplainable miracles in the NICU, the odds were finally with us that Bennett would survive and come home with us. Our hearts were overjoyed that there was a discharge plan that would kick into effect after he was off oxygen and able to drink from a bottle on his own. We did not know when that would happen, but it thrilled us that there was a viable plan for discharge. What knocked the wind out of us was that Bennett had experienced massive brain damage resulting from a lack of oxygen to his brain on the last day of ECMO (per the daily brain scans). He was given a cerebral palsy diagnosis on the fortieth day of his NICU stay, and the future was one big blank, previously white, now a murky gray canvas full of unknowns and ambiguity.

After listening to the MRI results, we drove home that day feeling shocked, sad, and confused. It felt like an entire new ending scene to a movie had been added to the script, but we were confused because we naïvely thought we already knew how it ended. We had chatted with the NICU social worker for a little while and she offered us some sincere advice, but there was nothing she could say in that moment to aid us. She encouraged us to go home and take some time to process his diagnosis, so we drove home while it was still light outside and walked up our old creaky wooden stairs to find a brown manila envelope waiting on our porch with the return label stating, "The White House."

We had no idea what was inside, so we numbly tore open the other mail, and then when we found a letter opener, we carefully opened the envelope and read a kind note dated September 19, 2007, from President George W. Bush, reading:

Dear Kelly and Travis:
Marv told me that Bennett is going through a tough time. Laura and I will keep him and your entire family in our thoughts and prayers. We know you are looking forward to bringing him home soon.
Best wishes and may God bless you.
Sincerely,
George W. Bush

Travis and I stood there reading the words on the White House stationery's cream cardstock and we were speechless. Receiving this letter on the very day that we were processing a difficult and devastating diagnosis, we did feel like we got a little hug from *up above* assuring us to keep trusting, keep believing, and keep hoping.

As humans we all instinctually have innate mechanisms for coping with trauma. In our case, our brains and hearts immediately tried to make sense of the broad spectrum of facts and feelings. *Thank God our baby is alive . . . he is so beautiful and perfect . . . he is so alert and knows the sound of our voices . . . he will be able to go home and sleep in his crib . . . he will be able to wear his clothes that are waiting for him . . . what will our lives look like with a son with severe brain damage?*

Late one evening after we had been given the cerebral palsy diagnosis and shared the information with our families, I sat next to my dad, Chris, near the hospital's elevator bank next to a soda machine. While I was growing up, my family had dear friends who had a grown son with cerebral palsy, who lived a joyful life in his wheelchair, and lived an incredible life well into his fifties. We knew that Bennett could live a full and wonderful life with cerebral palsy, but we also knew from firsthand observations that a lot is required to care for a person unable to care for themselves. As I gulped down tears in the glow of the soda machine, I said, "I am just so sad for Travis. I want him to have a son who can play basketball with him, throw him a baseball, and just wrestle around with. What if Bennett will never be able to play with him?" My dad, probably completely caught off guard with such raw grief, replied, "Oh, Kel, Bennett is going to play basketball and do all those things with Travis. We just have to keep praying and believe." The image of a blond-haired, blue-eyed boy one day dribbling a basketball with his daddy was the tangible hope I was holding on to in that moment.

CHAPTER 9

Preparing to Bring Bennett Home

"The greatest strength is the spirit of endurance."
— Lailah Gifty Akita

THERE WERE TWO milestones that we needed to meet for Bennett to be allowed to come home from the hospital. He had to drink from a bottle in order to gain weight daily, based on the neonatologist's determined amount, and he had to be weaned from the oxygen that he was reliant on. The oxygen reliance was slowly improving, but while intubated, Bennett could not drink from a bottle. He had been fed nutrients via a tube that went through his nostril and down the back of his throat so he had had no practice in drinking from a bottle. This tended to be a big stumbling block for a lot of NICU babies, especially for those who experienced acid reflux (which Bennett had), so we knew we had another large hurdle to overcome.

Soon after Bennett's MRI result his breathing tube was removed from his throat, and a nightmare CPAP mask experience commenced. These were crazy-tense days in the NICU as Bennett's oxygen levels would be stable in the 90s one minute (mid- to high 90s were considered acceptable), and then he could plummet down to the 50s in the blink of an eye. We were constantly scared that he would have to be intubated again (or even worse, have a tracheotomy placed), so the days were long as he absolutely hated the mask over his face (with strong air blowing in his nostrils). He basically screamed nearly the entire time he was on the CPAP machine. Thankfully the doctors created the order and he was finally given a nasal cannula for oxygen administration. The nasal cannula was a huge step for multiple reasons, mostly because if he required oxygen for a prolonged time he could go home with a nasal cannula and oxygen. We were more and more anxious to get our baby home, and any step closer to home was considered a big win.

A few days following his nasal cannula, I walked into the NICU and the nurse instructed me to go to the huge freezer where I had been placing the bags of my pumped breast milk. She told me that we were going to thaw out a bag and that I would be feeding Bennett via bottle that day. *Excuse me, what?* The speech therapists had come by to do a consultation, and they felt he was ready to try a bottle. After more than forty days of intubation, he was at risk for an oral aversion (a rejection of any nipple placed in his mouth), so the sooner we introduced the bottle, and kept doing so consistently, the better the chances were for his natural sucking reflexes to suck down the milk. I watched the nurse place the plastic bag full of breast milk into a plastic canister full of hot water to thaw it out for a few minutes, watched her pour my milk into a small bottle, screw on the nipple, and hand it over to me.

For many mothers, a core desire is the ability to feed their child. I was one of those mothers who had dreamed of that moment, and finally hope was realized. I held Bennett in my arms, his nasal cannula still in his nostrils, and his big blue eyes staring up at me. I placed the tip of the nipple gently into his mouth, and immediately he used that little tongue to shove the nipple right out of his mouth. After a few more gentle attempts and a few drops of the sweet breast milk placed on his tongue, he finally started to suck the nipple, swallowed the milk, and my maternal longing had been fulfilled.

We worked hard in the coming days and weeks to get Bennett to drink a bottle. When I say "we" I mean me, Travis, grandmas, Travis's sister Meredith, all the nurses, speech therapists, and anyone else who had ever had success getting a Georgetown NICU baby to drink a bottle. It literally took a village. Bennett would drink some breast milk from the bottle, but he would never finish the number of ounces that the doctors were wanting him to drink, so his feeding tube stayed in his nose. He was eventually discharged from the NICU with the tube, and his eating challenges were its own beast that we'd wrestle with for his entire first year and a half of life.

Before we knew it, Bennett was requiring less and less oxygen support. The NICU fellow who had originally told us, "Your baby is drowning; we do not expect him to survive" was now telling us that Bennett would have chronic lung disease for up to seven years, asthmatic symptoms being very possible, but after that his lungs had a high probability of being fully restored. Much to our surprise, one day we walked up to Bennett's crib to visit him and his nasal cannula had been removed. For the first time ever we saw our son's full face with no plastic tubing obstructing his big beautiful eyes (those thick lashes!), perfect nose, and rosy cheeks.

The sight of his precious face took my breath away. *Hey there, handsome little fella.* His nurse assigned to him that day reported, "Today we are trying him out on room air and so far he is doing fantastic." We were cautiously optimistic as we knew that NICU life many times included three steps forward, two steps back; but to think that we had gone from ECMO to room air was stunning to say the least. As it sunk in that we were so close to going home (we knew we could bring him home with his feeding tube to help supplement the nutrients he did not ingest by mouth), the excitement, linked with many unknowns, was overwhelming. How much equipment would be coming home with us? How many prescriptions, how many times a day, would we be administering? Would he need to come home with a heart monitor and oxygen?

All of the logistics concerns were instantly put on the back burners of our minds the day that we learned that a case of MRSA was in the NICU. Methicillin-resistant Staphylococcus aureus (MRSA) is a bacterium that causes infections in different parts of the body. It's tougher to treat than most strains of staphylococcus aureus, or staph, because it's resistant to some commonly used antibiotics. It is common knowledge that infection is one of the highest risks of staying in a hospital, so after sixty days in the NICU, being stable on room air and working to drink a bottle, we felt the walls were closing in on us. We could not make peace with the fact that Bennett had survived all that he had, but now the risk of MRSA taking his life was three cribs away from him. We were grateful that baby was placed in isolation (and survived), and Bennett was placed in a room that was the last "stop on the train" before going home. Within days we heard the best news of our parental journey thus far: It was finally time to bring our baby home. After nearly seventy days in the NICU, facing death and overcoming numerous obstacles, it appeared that Bennett was indeed coming home.

Most NICUs have a policy saying that for parents to prepare for what life will be like at home, you are expected to "room in" at the hospital with your baby the night before your baby is being discharged. Our night had finally come. The NICU team had been excited to announce to us that the night was finally here, and we were overjoyed that Bennett's NICU journey was coming to an end. On Friday, October 26, 2007, we nervously entered our hospital room for the night and waited for the nurses to bring Bennett in to us. Two nurses wheeled his crib into our room, gave us a few instructions regarding his feeding pump, meds schedule, and heart monitor tips, gave us smiles and hugs, and closed the door. We breathed a huge sigh of relief. We were finally together, alone, as our little family of three. We took a moment to savor this sweet moment, and then the screaming began. Bennett looked around, was overwhelmed with it all, and proceeded to scream on and off for the rest of the night. We slept zero hours, had a few check-ins from the nurses (but they could not calm him) and by the wee hours of the morning as we reported back to the charge nurse what was going on, she smiled and said, "Yes, that has been his nightly routine here in the NICU too." It had been reported to us that some nurses, exhausted caring for him at night, would request a doctor's order to give him morphine to calm his nerves. Now we understood why.

Travis and I stumbled out of the NICU to the parking garage just after sunrise, completely exhausted and shaken. Bennett was tucked back into his NICU area while we were sent home to try and get some rest. We were starving and depleted, so we drove straight to a local McDonald's and self-medicated with coffee, juice, and pancakes. Quite frankly, we were terrified that the previous night was going to be our new nightly routine and were trying to somehow find a way to prepare ourselves for this new normal. We went straight home, crashed for a long nap, woke up, showered, and headed to a local French café for our last quiet meal with just the two of us.

As we walked to the café around the corner from our house, I recall breathing in the cool fall air and watching the leaves blow up and down the busy street with each gust of wind. It was the end of October, my most favorite time of year. The summer humidity had rolled out, and the cool, dry air was honey to my battered soul. As Travis and I sat across the small table from each other, trying intentionally to swallow gulps of food, my body shook with fear. I could not force food down a throat that had no appetite. I did not know what the coming days held, but my gut instinct was telling me it was going to be more challenging and harder than I could even fathom. His nonstop screaming would continue, I would be exhausted keeping up with around-the-clock meds and breathing treatments, the heart monitor would be going off at random times, and his acid reflux and oral aversion would be a constant stress as we tried to feed him the nutrients he so desperately needed for healing. Even so, we sat there in those two wobbly café chairs, trying to force smiles and stay positive as we reflected on the seventy days in the NICU—all the miracles and memorable moments—while tears ran down my cheeks onto my croissant wrapper. *Hope, I need you.*

CHAPTER 10
Bennett Comes Home

"For My thoughts are not your thoughts,
neither are your ways My ways,' declares the Lord."
— Isaiah 55:8

WE PULLED UP to the NICU with our brand-new infant car seat, facing backwards of course, safely strapped in the back seat of our car and were greeted by my parents waiting for us anxiously. They were beyond eager to photograph and video the much-awaited moment of bringing our son home seventy days post-birth. We all nervously rode the elevator up to the third floor one last time, where Bennett was waiting for us all dressed in an adorable blue, green, and gray sweater onesie I had picked out—my favorite outfit for him, one I had envisioned bringing him home in. That day had finally come, and now we got to share it with family, doctors, respiratory therapists, receptionists, as well as several of our favorite nurses. They had all grown to love our baby and it was very fitting for us all to gather together in this moment.

My dad, Chris, owned an American flag that had flown over the US Capitol, so we presented it to the Georgetown NICU medical team as a thank-you for all they had done to save Bennett's life and care for him with such dedication. Many tears were shed as I read out loud the letter presented with the flag, and as Travis gave a few short words of gratitude. We looked into the teary eyes of our nurses, who had become like sisters to us, and fumbled over words of thanks as we said goodbye to the neonatologists, fellows, respiratory therapists, techs, and administrative staff. The rush of emotion and fluster of feelings was a juxtaposition that left us feeling extremely inept about finding a way to properly thank this group of people.

Nurse Ashley's reflections upon our leaving the NICU

I have truly never been so excited to go in to work on a day off as I was the day I went in to see Bennett leave the NICU with his parents. The thought of that day still gives me chills.

I held Bennett in my arms as Travis pushed us in a wheelchair down to the circle drive that we had walked on every day for the past seventy days. It was the same circle drive where we parked on the devastating day that I was discharged from the hospital without my baby—Travis then pulling away from the curb with me barely holding myself together as I tried not to have my milk letdown come gushing through my shirt as my body primally longed for my baby. We later were told that our parents and siblings stood along that brown brick wall along the circle drive holding back their own tears, disbelief, and deep grief for us as we were discharged without him.

Yet on this chilly fall day in October we drove home together, finally, as our family of three, and Travis will tell you he was an absolute nervous wreck with each turn. Bennett had been given a calming medication right before we left the NICU, so he did not scream, but, rather, his big eyes looked up at the large foreign shapes as we passed the old tree-lined streets of Northwest D.C. Our baby boy was more than two months old, and he had never seen a tree. The historic, sprawling oak trees of Northwest D.C. are definitely worthy of admiration, and Bennett seemed to take in each new shape as we drove. We pulled up to the little blue house and were delighted to see a large sign across the small and cozy front porch: "WELCOME HOME BENNETT MITCHELL SPECK." Our dream had come true. Our son was finally home.

Travis held Bennett tightly as we entered our house, the cold fall air hitting our baby's face for the first time. A crocheted blue and white blanket, made with love by his grandmother, covered him up. Grandpa documented each moment via video as Travis gave Bennett a short tour of his new home and I worked quickly to set up his medications and positioned his heart monitor and the feeding pump next to his crib. Soon thereafter Bennett did begin to fuss, so the grandparents waved goodbye and let us have time to get settled and soak in the gravity of this moment. Bennett was home and we were holding him in our arms, which numerous times throughout the past two months we thought would never happen. In fact, there were many dark nights when we had each, at different times, convinced ourselves quite frankly that it was not ever going to happen. We had prayed and begged God to save Bennett, and we both sincerely believed with all our hearts in the saving God of the universe. We had each learned from a very young age the Bible verse that says, "Ask and it will be given to you; seek and you will find; knock and the door will be opened to you. For everyone who asks, receives; the one who seeks, finds; and to the one who knocks, the door will be opened" (Matthew 7:7-8).

That said, we also knew in a very real way that God does not always answer prayers exactly the way that His believers request of Him. Sometimes His answer is "No" or "Later" or "Soon" or "Trust Me" even when we are desperately begging for a different outcome. Until we were standing with Bennett in our arms inside the little blue house, we did not claim to know what God's plan was. He was discharged with a very grim and real prognosis explained to us. He had cerebral palsy, with significant brain damage that most likely would result in a seizure disorder. He might not sit, stand, walk, or talk. Everyone tried to be encouraging and end with positive thoughts: "But you never know! Kids are resilient and have an amazing way of surprising us."

One NICU neonatologist actually took us aside and quietly told us she had seen "worse" MRIs for kids who ended up being very high-functioning and capable. There was no way to make sense of all that had happened in the NICU, nor could we attempt to know what God was planning to do with the life of Bennett Speck. We had not had a typical NICU experience involving birth, time spent in the NICU, complications, triumphs, and a discharge home with a healthy baby.

There were losses felt deep in our core, a lot to grieve (alongside some very significant "wins"), and a ten-week-old miracle boy belonging to two very weary yet grateful parents. We had been two structured, hard-working planners who thought we had some control over our family's life. We were quickly learning that we had very little control in this journey we call life. We were also being forced to accept that we were going to have to take each day as it came, pivoting as needed for the unknown road that lay ahead.

CHAPTER 11

Dig Deep (Life at Home After the NICU)

"Maybe you are searching among the branches
for what only appears in the roots. "
— Rumi

ENNETT WAS DRINKING from a bottle when he was discharged from the NICU, but he was not drinking enough ounces deemed acceptable by the doctors. They had specific calorie calculations as to how much he should be ingesting each day, and he rarely met their goals. As much as we did not want to go home with a feeding tube, Bennett was discharged with a nasogastric (NG) tube. An NG tube is a very narrow tube that runs through a nostril and down the back of one's throat. We connected his feeding pump to the end of the NG tube to ensure the proper amount of food entered his body each day, at a very slow rate. The slow feeding rate was extremely crucial as he had terrible acid reflux due to over forty days of intubation. If the pump's rate was too high, or he was jostled too much, it was a foregone conclusion that projectile vomiting (a.k.a. "milk bath") was imminent.

Bennett required the administration of seven different medications, was going through morphine withdrawal, and he screamed *a lot* for most of his waking hours. That is not an over-exaggeration. For all we know he had a raging migraine headache in addition to horrible drug withdrawals. His poor little sensory system could not handle the sound of a freezer door being shut or even a startling noise on the television. We would feed him, change his diaper, swaddle him, and sit in the glider rocking him while he screamed at the top of his lungs. We tried turning off the light, turning on the light, standing up and bouncing up and down, but nothing worked. Bennett would eventually completely wear himself out from screaming. He would pass out asleep, we would lay him down in his crib, administer his medications, turn on his feeding pump, and then both collapse into bed in emotional and physical exhaustion.

There were not a lot of words spoken between us during those first few days or nights after we brought Bennett home from the hospital. Our moms had each offered to help us, but we felt deeply that we had to figure out how to care for Bennett on our own. We both had fresh memories of our "rooming in" nightmare at the hospital; we had to see if it was just as challenging at home. Travis had taken the week off from work after bringing Bennett home, so we prepared ourselves to hunker down to figure this out together.

The first week home consisted of our scarfing down food here and there, trying to get Bennett to drink a bottle, practicing his "tummy time" while he wailed, attempting to get him down for a nap, or walking him around attached to our bodies in the baby carrier attempting to soothe him. By nightfall, as Travis and I collapsed into bed together, some nights we lay facing opposite directions, most likely crying. On other nights, we simply hugged each other tightly, and said not a word. We both knew in our hearts that we had to *dig deep*. We had to persevere as we had never persevered before. Bennett could not help it. He could not help that the giant world was completely overwhelming to him every second that his eyes were open.

It was sobering to simply look at the facts of all that was happening in Bennett's little body: morphine withdrawal, severe acid reflux causing his spine to arch in pain, and sensory overload. None of this was his fault. And yet we were forced to find new coping mechanisms for ourselves to deal with this new constant level of stress, crisis, and 24/7 care for a medically fragile child. Each day for me involved waking up with a huge knot in my stomach, zero appetite, with no ability to grocery shop, think straight, or go anywhere. To cope with all of this, I would simply strive to grab a hot shower at some point during the day to allow myself to breathe, cry, and attempt to reset. The days were bearable, but as the autumn sun began to set, the darkness swallowed up our home. The night shadows consisted of pacing, rocking, and bouncing a screaming baby while two adults shuffled through the house numbly responding to this new normal.

Looking back, Travis and I should have accepted help from our mothers that first week. That week was so hard, so miserable, and so taxing. We each lost several pounds because there was no quiet moment to eat and we rarely had appetites, even though friends brought us dinner every night. We were scared to death, unsure how we could physically sustain this insanity, but just kept doing what we knew we had to do.

Three days after discharge from the NICU, Bennett had to be checked out by a pediatrician at Georgetown. We went into the appointment hopeful and proud that we had successfully cared for our fragile infant at home on our own. Unfortunately, the appointment turned out to be a nightmare experience. Following a long wait in the crowded waiting room, the stoic doctor told us that Bennett appeared to be doing well post-discharge, but he added that our baby's development was not typical and we "should not expect a normal life." We left the appointment feeling discouraged, shaken, and socked in the gut once more.

Travis went to get our car from the parking garage while I dropped off Bennett's prescription for morphine at the hospital pharmacy; he was still being weaned off of this narcotic. I then waited, with Bennett in his car seat, in the lobby of the building, looking out the window at the gray, gloomy, and rainy day outside. It was clear that the pharmacy was running behind, so we were going to have to wait a while. Unfortunately, I also knew that Bennett would be waking up and screaming at any moment, so I began to sweat.

Bennett did indeed wake up a few moments later. His eyes opened, he started looking around, and I know he was thinking, "Where in the world am I?" I tried to feed him, but he did not want the bottle; thus his crying began. He would take a few sips of his bottle, but then he would wail and wail. As I sat there nervously looking out the window, I was grateful to soon see Travis pulling up. I quickly picked up Bennett's car-seat carrier, covered it with a blanket, and headed out into the rain. I hurriedly locked Bennett's car seat into the back seat of the car and told Travis that I had to go back in to get his morphine prescription. Travis's stressed face informed me to hurry. Our car was not supposed to stay parked outside the building, so Travis had to circle the building amidst a disastrous construction zone as I ran back into the pharmacy in the lobby. I immediately walked up to the counter to see if they could estimate when the prescription would be ready. I will never forget the way that the pharmacy employee asked me, "Morphine for a baby? What baby needs morphine?" Due to the controlled substance that it is, I immediately felt all the eyes in the pharmacy on me, as though I was being suspected of trying to illegally get a prescription for morphine. I was filled with shame, but that shame quickly turned to anger as I replied, "It is for my baby who just got discharged from the NICU after spending sixteen days on ECMO and forty days of intubation. If you do not believe me, feel free to call up there right now and a neonatologist will be happy to vet my story." She looked annoyed, but filled the prescription, checked me out, and in tears I walked to the car. As Travis finally circled around and pulled up the car, I found a stressed-out dad. Bennett was screaming, I was crying, and that miserable, rainy October day was a day I hoped so badly I would one day forget.

Hospital and specialist bills began to show up in our mailbox, and each day that we checked our mail we braced ourselves for the huge bill. We had incredible health insurance through my job at the time, but estimating the astronomical costs associated with seventy days in the NICU left us expecting we would be receiving bill(s) capable of wiping out our savings account. Upon our NICU discharge, it soon came to our attention that our health insurance would not pay for full-time home nursing. Upon hearing the news, believe it or not, we were not all that upset. There was simply too much happening. There had been endless lists of logistics to sort out prior to Bennett's discharge from the NICU. We had to have oxygen at home in case his oxygen levels tanked. We had a heart monitor, a feeding pump, and a nebulizer delivered to our house to ensure we had all the supports he needed. We had been trained well by his NICU nurses, and frankly we felt it was our responsibility (and privilege) to care for our son.

Yet surprisingly, due to the religious (Catholic) foundation of Georgetown University, the hospital had relationships with certain nursing agencies employing medically trained nuns who worked for discounted fees. We were delighted to find out that we actually did have a home nursing option, so we had agreed to have a one-hour weekly visit from one of the religious women's nursing agencies. Yet once we arrived home and the tornado of daily life caring for Bennett began, I simply forgot to expect a visit from a nurse.

One beautiful crisp, sunny, fall afternoon I heard a knock on our red door as I was walking Bennett around the house, trying to keep him from crying. Travis had just returned to his full-time job, so I was holding Bennett when I opened the door to find a petite African nurse in her habit smiling back at me. I was stunned and asked, "Can I help you?" She smiled a big and beautiful grin and replied, "I am Nurse Ann and I have been sent to help you with your baby." I stood completely baffled (maybe it was the habit she wore?), but the baby started to scream, so in a gesture of desperation I invited Nurse Ann in. It was her endearing smile and the twinkle in her eyes that told me she was trustworthy. She came in, washed her hands, opened her arms and asked, "May I hold him?" My mothers' instinct told me she was safe, and my pure exhaustion permitted me to hand Bennett over to her.

On that first day Nurse Ann insisted that I do whatever I needed to do while she watched him. Her kind help had come so unexpectedly I simply asked if I could take a shower. I prepared a bottle for Bennett and told her that he might drink it, or he might get agitated and start screaming. She asked why he was so unhappy, and I told her that we did not know. "The doctors think he is still withdrawing from morphine from his time on ECMO."

After I was in the shower, I heard Bennett's wails cranking up, and yet over the wails I heard a soprano-toned joyous voice bellowing, "Jesus, I love You! Jesus, I love You!" I knew he was in holy hands, so I took the opportunity to close my eyes and have a moment to weep while the water poured over my exhausted, drained body. In the shadow of our grief, we were sent an angel in the form of an African Catholic nun, Nurse Ann.

Nurse Ann's smile lit up the room, her voice was like a songbird's, and her weekly visits became a gift to our family. Nurse Ann's joy was contagious amidst our daily intensity and stress caring for Bennett. Any time she was stressed while attending to Bennett (usually involving re-inserting his NG tube up his nostril and down his throat), she chanted "Jesus, I love You" over and over. In our challenging and lonely days of figuring out how best to care for Bennett, we had been sent an incredible gift wrapped in a habit. Hope was near.

CHAPTER 12
Screaming and Moving

"You can buy a bed, but you cannot buy rest."
— Rick Wilkerson, Jr.

ACH NIGHT THAT Travis came home from work, he came home to more than five hours of Bennett's screaming until finally Bennett would pass out and sleep. We gulped down some form of dinner and tried to watch a little television together, but soon fell into bed completely exhausted ourselves. It was not what I had envisioned life would be like as a family of three. I had daydreamed of after-work family walks down our favorite tree-lined streets of Chevy Chase, Bennett resting against my chest in a baby carrier, and Travis and I holding hands as we strolled. We attempted such a family walk once or twice, but quickly ended up home after Bennett's wailing started and neighbors gave us awkward, bewildered stares. Nothing was easy. Nothing was normal. Nothing was predictable. Every simple task seemed difficult and exhausting.

Yet amidst the hard, there was still a lot of good. We had local friends dropping off dinners to us regularly, our moms came to help us with Bennett for a week each, and dear friends came through town from far-off states to make sure we were doing okay. A particularly caring older man from our church took the time to drive to our little blue house from his house miles away in the suburbs to meet Bennett, visit with us, pray with us, drop off a small stuffed toy lion, and to encourage us that Bennett was a fighter like a little ferocious lion. We were extremely touched by such kind and thoughtful gestures.

Travis's thirtieth birthday was soon approaching, Internet shopping was not a real thing yet, and knowing we could not have any form of a party, I desperately wanted to get him a gift. When the day of his birthday arrived, I strapped Bennett to my chest in his carrier, grabbed a bottle for backup, and walked down the street to a local department store. We rode up several escalators as I gave myself a pep talk to prepare for this first shopping outing. *We can do this, Bennett. Daddy deserves a birthday gift from us.* When we got into the store, I grabbed the first three things I saw that I thought Travis might like and headed for the checkout. Bennett started to fuss, so I stuck the bottle in his mouth, paid the cashier, grabbed the bag, and down the escalator we headed. This small triumph symbolized a big moment for me. It showed me I could find ways to still accomplish small tasks amidst this new intense normal. It was not pretty, and I probably looked like a frazzled crazy person, but that day showed me that I could leave my house. Bennett screamed the entire walk home down the tree-lined street of Northwest D.C., but I walked with my chin up and a great sense of achievement.

It quickly became clear that I could not return to my full-time job as my maternity leave was coming to a close. Ten of the twelve weeks I had spent visiting my baby in the hospital, with the last two weeks at home spent attempting to soothe a screaming baby. There was no nanny that we could hire to pass the baton to. I knew in my heart that I had to let my firm know that I could not return to my job, and Travis completely supported that decision. I made that very difficult call and they were completely understanding. It was both a difficult and an easy decision to make for me at the time. My baby needed me, my husband was able to work to pay our bills, and therefore my career needed to take an indefinite pause. I could not look to the future and deduce what this might mean for future work opportunities; instead I remember hanging up the phone (while sitting in the only quiet corner of our little blue house), and letting a few tears roll down my cheeks as the gravity of what I just did sank in.

As my mom, Kathy, saw the intensity of our daily lives with Bennett, one day she casually told us, "If you need help, please know that you are always welcome to move in with me." My parents had been divorced for five years, she lived alone in a three-bedroom townhouse in Virginia, and she worked full-time as a school social worker. We initially politely said, "Thanks so much for the offer, Mom, but we are fine. Surely things will start to get easier." Yet a week or so later, desperate times called for desperate measures, and Travis asked my mom if it would be okay if we moved in with her. She was surprised yet thrilled, and we started making plans to move to Virginia. We had been told that children's early intervention services were fantastic in her county in Northern Virginia, so we were excited to cross the Potomac River. It was not difficult to leave Washington, D.C., even though we had shared a lot of wonderful memories over the past four years. We loved the energy surrounding the city, restaurants, parks, and culture there, but the buzz of the city did not outweigh the traumatic experiences lived there, so it was time to move on.

Travis arranged for friends to come load up our boxes and furniture into a rented truck, I oversaw caring for Bennett, and he eagerly moved us to Virginia in early December of 2007. Moving to Virginia increased Travis's work commute significantly and caused us to find new doctors for Bennett, but in our hearts we knew that we needed more help and support with our daily life. The thought of my mom willing to cook a dinner for us or hold a screaming baby every now and then brought a rush of relief over us. We had tried hard to manage the chaos, but it was more than clear that we needed help.

Travis's sister and brother-in-law had flown up from Tennessee to help us move in with my mom the first weekend of December 2007. Somehow, we had thrown all our belongings into boxes, and a team of family and friends got our boxes and furniture put into trucks and unloaded at my mom's house. Bennett spent the day somewhat calm with my mom in her living room while we bustled around her townhouse, trying to make all our items "fit" among her belongings. We excitedly bought a new TV for her basement so we could watch the SEC Championship football game that day. We worked all day to get all the boxes and furniture settled in time for kickoff. We ordered pizzas to thank everyone and sat down excitedly to watch the game. It almost felt "normal." Yet just as the sun was setting, Bennett became agitated, and I spent the rest of the evening rocking him and trying to settle him in his new nursery. It may sound as though he suffered from a hard case of colic, and perhaps that is all it was. He was our first baby, so we had no frame of reference. If so, it felt like colic on monster-truck-sized steroids.

Once we were settled at my mom's house, Bennett's night screaming continued to crank up about 8 p.m. and went on until he finally fell asleep around midnight or one o'clock in the morning. To try to soothe him, I held him in my arms and rocked him in the glider; I stood up and bounced him; I swayed him back and forth giving him "white noise" by saying "Shhhh" near his little ears. We would swaddle him up tight and I would offer him the bottle, but usually he had no interest in it. When nothing else worked, I laid him down in his crib, surrounded by his small stuffed animal friends, to see if he simply did not want to be held or perhaps might be more comfortable lying flat with less stimulation.

In those moments when he was lying in the crib swaddled up,

screaming continuously, sadness poured over me that I was not able to soothe my baby. Bennett would not take a pacifier and was not able to bring his hands to his mouth, so sucking his thumb was not an option either. Each night it was a grueling experience, and yet I was completely committed to the task because Travis and my mom both had to go to work each day. *I am his mom. It is a miracle that he is alive to scream this much. I know deep within my soul that there is no place else I am supposed to be than with my baby as he screams. This is what mothers do. None of this is his fault.*

Each evening before going to bed, Travis would come in, check on us, hold his son before going to bed, and give him (and me) a goodnight kiss. But Bennett the night owl was just gearing up for the night. My mom tells the story that one night well after midnight she got up from her bed to use the restroom, peeked in at Bennett's room, and found Bennett asleep in his crib with me lying on the royal-blue carpet right next to him in a deep sleep. She did not wake me as she knew there was a chance the slightest noise could wake him, which would then lead to another one to three hours of screaming. Those nights were grueling and arduous to say the least.

I can still remember almost every detail of Bennett's small nursery at my mom's house. His white crib fit perfectly in the corner, next to a matching white bookcase filled with baby books that we would read him. He did love any book that had noises like a mooing cow or a snorting pig. We slowly rocked him in the glider facing the bookcase during the day and early evening, and he would be calm for small periods of time. But then, as the sun went down, darkness filled the room except for the light of the small night light shining down at the royal blue carpet. It almost felt as if we were wrestling with evil spirits during those nights in the nursery. Some nights we tried keeping the lights on to see if that would help, but nothing improved. Bennett screamed continuously, with a look of pure fear as we held him close, covered him in kisses, prayed continuously, and begged God to make it stop. As all parents can attest, there is no greater pain than watching our kids suffer with the feeling of complete helplessness, unable to take the pain from them.

Travis and I have been extremely fortunate to have had incredible mentors in our lives. One of those mentors for me is a man named Bob Roth, whom I met while in my high-school youth group at church. He and his wife were newly married, and he had experienced an intentional faith journey by researching all the faiths and denominations available until he landed at the church that I grew up attending. Bob's education had previously taken him to graduate school at the University of Virginia, where he studied Russian Studies, and later became an FBI agent in March 1996. During the time that Bob was working to get into the FBI, he volunteered with our church youth group, teaching religious classes about his journey to his faith, and even chaperoned our youth group mission trip to an orphanage in Honduras.

I was fortunate enough to be on that mission trip to Honduras, and watching Bob's work ethic, heart for God, and love for his wife, whom he called every time he could find a pay phone, were ingrained in my mind. Bob was a man of integrity and character. If Bob said something, he meant every word. If he gave you advice, it was coming from a place of deep concern and was worth listening to. When I headed off to the University of Virginia for my first year of college, he encouraged me to spend more time at the church on Rugby Road than the fraternity houses on the other end of Rugby Road. He was always looking out for my best interests, and my favorite advice he ever gave me is, "The shortest distance between two points is a straight line." The "straight line" might not be the easiest way; in fact it may be the most challenging or hardest way, but based on my experiences, I think Bob was on to something.

Prior to Bennett's birth, in 2003 we began attending the same church in which we had married in 2000. Bob and his wife Tresa had since had five children, amidst busy careers. Their beautiful family was a pillar in our faith community and we loved visiting with them any chance that we could. I recall seeing Tresa one day in passing as she held her youngest toddler son on her hip. I smiled when I saw her and exclaimed, "You guys are amazing, Tresa! How do you do it?" I stood in awe of them as we were starting to long for our first child, having busy and promising careers ourselves. With her big stunning smile and twinkle in her eyes, Tresa replied, "I don't know about amazing, more like crazy!" And with that she held her son on her hip and chased her other son down the hall, her strong legs striding in her black pumps. Bob and Tresa's love for each other, their family, their church, their community, and their country, are hard to put into words. I will let the FBI website tell you more:

On the morning of September 11, 2001, American Airlines Flight 77 was commandeered by terrorists and crashed into the Pentagon, penetrating the building's five rings. A 200-foot fireball rose above the building engulfing the surrounding area in smoke, and a 100-foot section of the Pentagon's outer ring collapsed less than an hour later. Supervisory Special Agent Robert Martin Roth was one of the first agents to arrive and immediately began assisting injured personnel and securing debris. The environment around the crash scene contained heavy smoke from burning aviation fuel and smoldering debris. Roth stayed on the scene for two weeks, working twelve-hour days, and spent considerable time in the impact area.

In October 2006, Roth was diagnosed with multiple myeloma, and he succumbed to his illness on March 16, 2008. Extensive research by the Centers for Disease Control and the National Institute for Occupational Safety and Health established sufficient evidence that Roth's exposure to the air in and around the Pentagon after the 9/11 attack either precipitated or accelerated his development of multiple myeloma.

Special Agent Roth was born in December 1963. He entered on duty with the FBI in March 1996.

Four nights before he died, Bob and Tresa called my mom's house and asked to speak to Travis. I remember my mom handing the phone to Travis, where Bob and Tresa together asked Travis to sing at Bob's funeral. I stood watching the conversation in tears. Bob and Tresa had attended Bennett's prayer vigil on August 25 and now Bob's life on earth was coming to an end. He was my most influential high school mentor and I was devastated.

I was devastated that Tresa was losing her husband and that his five children were losing their dad much too young. Bob was a hero to me and many others. I was equally devastated that because of the exhaustion and all-consuming energy of caring for Bennett, I had not spent any time reaching out to them to offer my love and support as they walked the grueling health journey with Bob as his time on this earth came to a close.

As Travis rocked Bennett in his glider in his room at Mom's house, he listened, spoke quietly with Bob and Tresa, and mapped out how they wanted the service to go while taking notes of the specific songs that were important to them. The conversation did not last long, but it was a conversation that we will never forget.

Bob died three days later, and his death was a blow to each of us, to our families, our entire church community, not to mention Bob's family, friends, and the FBI. His funeral was the first occasion for which I left Bennett with anyone (thank God for Nurse Ashley, his NICU nurse). Travis somehow held it together and sang beautifully as he looked out at the large crowd, including a sizeable group of FBI agents and staff, with many well-known FBI officials in attendance.

Every pew in the church was full, standing room only, and somehow Travis mustered the composure to honor the commitment that he made to Bob by singing the meaningful songs of faith that Bob had requested. I sat sobbing in the pew as I watched Tresa walk down the middle aisle with her five young children following in a line behind her. I continued to weep, along with hundreds of others, throughout the service as I tried to process the deep loss the world was experiencing because of the loss of our dear friend, Special Agent, and man of God, Bob Roth.

Bennett stops crying

Just before Bob's death, around the time of the Super Bowl 2008, Bennett's nightly screaming sessions diminished. He was around six months old, and instead of screaming until one or two o'clock in the morning, he found that he enjoyed lying in his crib to look at his new favorite Fisher-Price Rainforest musical mobile. It had brightly colored rainforest animals who rotated around in circles while music played, and he found this to be quite exciting. It was right around this time that he would start kicking his legs when excited about something. Each kick which he initiated filled us with joy. Speaking of joy, one night Travis was giving him a bath in a baby tub, inside the big bathtub, and as Travis poured the water over his little belly to wash off the bubbles, Bennett let out the biggest belly laugh we had ever heard. I had read in a book that if your baby laughed, that meant that part of their brain was processing emotion, which was an encouraging sign. We did not get a lot of laughs, but certain animal noises in his books, and other random noises, would bring about the belly laugh that we lived for.

There were kicks and giggles, but Bennett still startled easily and had a very strong startle reflex that would bring his arms stretched out above his head, pulsating his arms. These startles could be triggered by closing the freezer door too loudly, dropping a utensil on the floor, or even a loud noise on the TV. Once the startle dissipated, he usually cried for a while. Soon after, we realized the startle and pulsating arms were actually small seizures taking place. This would begin our journey into the world of neurology and a diagnosis of seizure disorder.

Three things that everyone had told us from the minute we were discharged from the NICU were "Early intervention is key. Children's brains are extremely malleable. Regeneration of brain pathways is very possible." A few weeks after we settled in at my mom's townhouse, I contacted the local Early Intervention services, and they were quick to come to us for an evaluation. It was clear that Bennett was significantly delayed in all aspects of "normal" infant development, so we were approved for physical therapy (PT), occupational therapy (OT), and speech therapy (to assist with feeding). I was extremely excited for professionals to guide me on how best to support Bennett in his development. During this time our goal was always to help Bennett to meet *his* greatest potential, not to wear him out (or ourselves) by chasing the chance of reaching "normal" or "typical"—whatever that means, anyway!

Home physical therapy soon began, and we worked every day on tummy time, sitting up assisted in a foam support chair, and reaching for toys. Through tons of reading, we had learned how humans develop. If a baby can sit, they can then stand and later walk. So for us, step one involved working on sitting up. Core strength was truly crucial to each goal that we had for Bennett. We worked on sitting up all day every day, amidst some tummy time, lying in his crib to see his favorite musical mobile, and tons of snuggles, of course. After months and months of physical therapy via the early intervention program, plus private physical therapy, we were not seeing any improvement in Bennett's sitting skills. We knew this was not the best news, but we kept working on weight bearing with his legs, hoping that over time our little miracle boy might continue to surprise us. We desperately hoped that he would one day walk, so we kept lifting prayers up, but also we worked on celebrating who Bennett was. By this point he was a chubby, smiley, delightful baby who brought us much joy. He had us all wrapped around his little clenched fists (which stayed clenched throughout the day due to his increased muscle tone from his cerebral palsy).

Bennett's first birthday was approaching, and we decided to both celebrate him and thank our community who had supported us each day of the past year. We had received so many prayers, gift cards, cards, gifts, and words of encouragement that had literally kept us going on some of our hardest days during that year. As a way to celebrate the miracle of a year of life with Bennett, we rented a picnic space at a local working farm, bought a bunch of snack food, and ordered a huge farm-themed cake. His farm-animal books with the mooing cows and snorting pigs had brought him such joy and giggles, what could be more fitting? We invited family and friends, and hoped that families could grab a snack, cake, and a balloon while enjoying the working farm. Bennett was not able to eat the cake nor could he handle being the center of attention—he pretty much wanted to be left alone in his stroller. Regardless, it was a memorable day of celebrating one year of life with Bennett, and we deeply appreciated all the friends and family who made the effort to come out and celebrate our miracle boy.

After turning one, Bennett's left eye began to creep inwards. This resulted from his cerebral palsy's "increased tone," which means his muscles were tighter/stiffer. Following the brain damage even the muscles in his eyes had tightened. As a result, Bennett soon won the family award for "First family member to get Botox!" We set up an appointment with a well-known pediatric ophthalmologist at Georgetown, and Bennett got Botox injections in his left eye muscles to attempt to relax the muscle that was pulling his eye inward. Following the Botox procedure, we did eye patching on the right eye (his "good eye") to try strengthening those left-eye muscles. We saw some good results and have continued patching through the years whenever we see that left eye creeping inwards. He did not have a stigmatism and therefore did not require glasses at that point.

Subsequent to Bennett's NICU discharge, we had somehow managed to get enough calories into Bennett by mouth. We combined breast milk with formula for added calories, and he had been gaining weight at a rate his pediatrician found acceptable. We were thrilled to have avoided a permanent gastric-tube surgery while he was in the NICU, but all that changed when Bennett, aged eighteen months, went cold turkey and stopped eating food by mouth. I clearly remember the last day that I sat on the couch to feed him a bottle. He drank it peacefully, and I was thankful for the calm way he fell asleep afterwards. Yet, for a reason we will never know, from that day onward he simply refused a bottle. Feeding him pureed baby foods was becoming more and more of a struggle as it usually caused coughing, gagging, or choking. We do not know exactly what happened or changed. Was it neurological? Was it acid reflux? Regardless, the sudden inability to eat by mouth was devastating.

Once Bennett stopped drinking a bottle, the NG tube was placed through his nostril and down his throat, and we knew it was time to adhere to the doctor's recommendation to place a permanent feeding tube, or g-tube, into Bennett's stomach. The night before Bennett's surgery at Children's National Hospital to place the g-tube, I felt very sad as I gazed at his bare stomach and stroked his creamy, baby-soft skin. I even took a picture of his stomach. I knew in my heart that once the tube was placed, it would be there permanently. We had worked hour by hour over eighteen months to get our son eating by mouth. We had performed multiple swallow studies in hospitals to try and figure out why eating was such a struggle, and yet all the efforts and tears had led us to this day. The swallow studies had discovered that he consistently aspirated food when he swallowed it, so the risk of developing pneumonia was too high to continue allowing food by mouth. I grieved his perfect bare belly, knowing a plastic "button" inserted into his abdomen would soon stay there indefinitely.

I had mixed feelings. I was grateful there was a medical intervention to sustain his life while allowing easy administration of medicines, and yet I felt the deep loss of him losing the ability to eat by mouth and all the joys and satisfaction and normalcy that come with that skill. He would most likely never enjoy the taste of our favorite local pizza, my mom's delectable baked goods, or Travis's mom's melt-in-your-mouth summer sweet corn. I took a few moments to feel this great loss, my dream of my firstborn child eating by mouth seeming to slip away like sand through my fingers. As his mother, the one who carried him inside my womb for nine months, with dreams for his life that looked very different than this, I took a few moments to grieve deeply for what was not. And here is what I learned: *It is okay to be in despair while feeling grateful; both emotions can co-exist.* My baby's stomach would most likely never again be free of a plastic tube, and I was sad about that. I am thankful that in addition to those feelings, I still had hope that this would make both his life and ours easier.

CHAPTER 13
Escaping to Tennessee

"Life touches everybody. Life will mess with you."
— Chad Veach

NOT LONG AFTER his first birthday and following Bennett's feeding-tube placement, we settled into new routines of feeding Bennett and caring for his physical needs. We could finally get medications and milk into him easily and efficiently via his feeding tube, but it could come back out just as quickly, in projectile vomit fashion. We ended up decreasing how much formula he took in with each feeding and added overnight slow feedings to allow him to get the volume of formula that he needed. Through trial and error, and with the guidance of doctors, we found a feeding schedule that worked with his body's ability to digest. We had no home nursing help at this time (and for years to follow), so each day was an adventure in getting food into the belly of a sweet boy via his two rookie parents doing our best. The smell of formula became a familiar scent because spit-ups were the new normal. His reflux in addition to the feeding-pump-volume experiments felt like never-ending episodes of whack-a-mole most days.

By this point we were still living with my mom in Virginia, which was blessing us in multiple ways, one of which was the ability to save for our first home. Following Bennett's first birthday, there was a swelling desire to settle down, buy our first house, and have some independence as a family of three. By this point Bennett was actually evolving into a happy baby. He would sometimes even gurgle down a few tastes of baby food, but for the most part he spent his days napping, working on the latest home physical therapy exercise recommended to us by therapists, and watching his beloved Fisher-Price Rainforest mobile in his crib while he kicked with glee.

Travis commuted to his job in Bethesda, Maryland from Northern Virginia along the Dulles Tollway. This forty-five-minute commute gave him time to think, zone out, and process his life at age thirty. I, too, had more than enough time to think while I stayed home with Bennett, took him to appointments, made an occasional drive-through trip to McDonald's, or hung out with him at home working on his developmental milestones. To be honest, it felt as if we were living in a nightmare, each hoping that one day we would wake up to realize that I was still pregnant, our baby was safe and sound inside of me, and we had a perfectly normal birth and newborn experience lying ahead of us. Our coping mechanisms were in overdrive as we tried our hardest to love each other, trust God, connect with our faith community whenever we could physically and emotionally show up, and try to make sense of this new life with seizure meds, feeding pumps, and endless medical supplies.

We soon realized Bennett could not grasp hold of a baby rattle, could not bring his hand to his face to suck a thumb or finger, nor bring his arms together at midline to hold a bottle or teething ring. Without these basic skills learned by most babies by ages two to four months old, I jarringly realized that our son had no way to self-soothe, entertain himself, or explore his world on his own. It hit me hard that we were going to be responsible for entertaining and soothing him every waking minute of his day for his entire life. Not to be dramatic, but this was undeniably a large responsibility, especially for a relatively alert child who had strong opinions (yet no ability to communicate what his needs and wants were). The weight of this reality is still one to this day that we wrestle with.

SEC college football (more specifically, University of Tennessee football) was a huge part of Travis's childhood and family, so in the late fall of 2008 I planned a weekend getaway for Travis to meet up with his cousins, both Auburn grads, at the Auburn versus Tennessee football game. Travis had always wanted to attend this game with his cousins. I surprised him by purchasing football and airplane tickets, and we had the weekend circled on our calendar. Travis was really looking forward to the weekend and I wanted nothing more than for him to get away from his heavy responsibilities. I wanted him to relax, laugh, have a beer with his cousins, and spend time enjoying a great college football game.

Unfortunately, as the week leading up to the game arrived, I could tell that Bennett was getting sick, and it was not just a small cold. His breathing got more and more labored while I kept praying that it would go away. By that Thursday morning I knew he needed to be seen by a doctor, so I made an appointment with our pediatrician. After the doctor assessed Bennett, she suspected that he was fighting a respiratory virus and needed to be seen at Children's Hospital for further testing and observation. I was devastated to have to phone Travis and let him know about this development. I begged him to keep his plans and go on to the game, but he refused. He told me there was no way he could have fun knowing Bennett was sick. I knew that I would feel the same way if I were in his shoes, but it was disappointing for both of us that he would be missing the game.

Travis cancelled the airplane flight, his cousins were notified, and we spent almost a week at the hospital nursing our sweet boy back to health by watching Bennett's sick lungs fight yet another virus, praying that he might rebound from it as he had done in the past. We had family, friends, and co-workers come to visit us in the hospital, which was incredibly kind and encouraging. When Bennett was not sedated, he was very agitated by the new environment. He had an IV in his arm and oxygen tubes in his nostrils, so we would each put our faces right up to his to sing, talk, and "sigh" our familiar noises into his ears to let him know we were there. I recall the nurses watching us and commenting on the ways we worked to soothe Bennett. Even they noticed that he was not able to soothe himself. He eventually made a full recovery, and we were discharged from the hospital and returned to "normal life." Yet after that hospitalization our hearts were heavier, we felt even more beat down, and it was hard to simply bounce back to life. The reality of the life we had was exhausting, each hospitalization adding a layer to our load.

We needed to get away. It all started to feel like too much. We needed wide open spaces to process our very real reality. We needed less traffic, less noise, less politics after more than a year of crisis after crisis: life support and MRIs in the NICU, to then realizing that a small cold for Bennett could turn into a six-day stay at Children's Hospital. The longings of our hearts whispered that we needed an escape, so we started talking about options. Travis had a secure federal government job, yet we had friends in Franklin, Tennessee who owned a house there while the husband commuted back and forth to Washington, D.C. Our friend stayed with his friend in D.C. during the work week. Could we do that too? My mom would keep an empty bedroom for Travis, and she welcomed the company. We wondered, is this crazy? Yes, it probably was. But at the time we had lost all equilibrium after a year of perpetual turmoil.

We both loved spending time visiting his family in Tennessee, and had dreamed of one day living there. Travis's family had a close friend who was an experienced realtor just south of Nashville. To see what kind of housing options were out there, we contacted the realtor. She began sending us housing options, and we eventually found a beautiful sprawling ranch house on half an acre of land. The yard was meticulously cared for, it had a rosebush trellis in the backyard, and simply looked like it was waiting for us to move in.

We quickly planned a weekend trip to Tennessee to look at the ranch house and several other homes, and that weekend confirmed that we wanted to follow our dream of settling there. Bennett's medical care would be transferable there as the local children's hospital had a strong reputation, and the medical industry was booming in Nashville. When we got home from our Tennessee trip, we quickly began talking to our realtor about drawing up an offer. She did, and after a few negotiations, we were official first-time homeowners. We closed on the house, were handed our first set of keys to a home we owned, and began packing up to chase after the dream of a quieter life located in the green rolling hills of Tennessee.

Saying goodbye to friends, family, and our faith community in Virginia was difficult. These people had walked with us through Bennett's birth, NICU stay, and his first year of life—the darkest time in both our lives. We were like a family loaded into a covered wagon heading west during the 1800s, seeking a new life. Not far from our Tennessee house was an old, large, red wooden barn settled at the bottom of a hill in a green pasture. After we moved in and traveled back and forth along the two-lane road in front of the barn, the sight of it instantly washed peace over me. It felt as if we were in our forever home, and I was prepared to be buried in the backyard.

In January 2009 Travis began his commuting routine of spending the weekends with us and hopping on a flight early on Monday to head back to Washington, D.C., to perform his work week. Even though he was young, in his early thirties, and up for the challenge, it was not an easy task. His willingness to travel across the southeastern United States weekly to give us a more peaceful life was a sacrifice for which I was (and still am) extremely grateful. During the weekdays while he was gone, I stayed busy with Bennett, taking him to physical, occupational, and feeding therapies at a new pediatric therapy center that had been recommended to us by our friend and realtor. Lucky for us it was a few miles from our home and was exactly what we needed as we worked on Bennett's developmental goals.

The therapists and staff at the pediatric therapy center there welcomed us with open arms and loving hearts. They even had an inclusive preschool program that Bennett ended up attending, so he could receive some socialization while being pulled out for therapies through the day. He struck up a particularly sweet friendship with a blond-haired blue-eyed "typical" little girl who would "mother" him by bringing him his favorite books and toys. Their friendship and a precious photo landed them in the marketing brochure for the center, because they personified everything that is beautiful about pediatric inclusive learning. Children see differences in each other, but their curiosity and grace toward those differences can be an example for us all.

This community was such a gift to us as the first place that we came into as a "special-needs family" seeking a place for our son to be accepted, celebrated, and find his "fit." There were no other school or daycare options for Bennett in the area, and as Travis's airfare expenses were piling up by the week, I was feeling the tug more and more to look for a part-time work option. The biggest hurdle was that I could work only if we had reliable childcare to nurture, care for, and give Bennett what he needed. The inclusive preschool was exactly that for him, and the days spent there with his teachers and therapists are some cherished memories for us. We still keep in touch with many of them to this day.

Our neighborhood was quiet and safe, so many evenings we spent hour after hour walking up and down the streets of our neighborhood. We waved at cars as they passed us, Bennett banging his most beloved "boom box" toy waiting for his favorite song to play one more time. It was on those quiet and lonely streets of Tennessee that my heart began to heal from the trauma of Bennett's birth. I had not done any deep post-traumatic stress counseling work after he was born because there simply was no time or energy for it. But by pushing his stroller up and down those asphalt streets, my thoughts freely flowed uninterrupted. I cried in the moments that I felt the weight of deep losses such as toddler play dates, "Mommy and me" music classes, or listening for his first words.

Nashville is known for many things, including a church on every corner. We had friends and family scattered at wonderful churches throughout the city, and after visiting several we found a lovely church that we regularly attended. We had a few friends there, some more acquaintances, and more than anything we felt the community there would be loving and accepting of Bennett, his needs, and our limitations. Immediately the warmth, love, and compassion oozed out of most everyone we met, and we looked forward to going to church together as a family of three, savoring the time we had Travis home with us.

Nashville is also known for its rolling hills, magnificent estate houses scattered along the countryside, and beautifully landscaped lush green yards. One particularly beautiful spring Sunday morning we had Bennett with us in the church service when he started to get irritated, as was his normal behavior anytime he wanted to either get moving or take a nap. We were nervously looking at each other, trying to decide which of us should take him out to walk him around, when a kind woman sitting behind us tapped me on the shoulder. Her kind eyes met mine, yet I still braced to hear from her a "Shhhh! He is very loud." Instead of a complaint, however, she smiled and asked if she could push him around in the church foyer. I was pleasantly surprised and recognized her as a mother of several young kids, so I figured she "got it" and nodded yes. She stood up, took the handles of Bennett's wheelchair stroller, and whisked him out the doors of the auditorium. We knew he was in good hands, so Travis and I were able to sit together to take a breath to enjoy a few quiet moments.

It was a remarkably kind gesture for this woman, basically a stranger to us, to see that Bennett was not "typical" or "normal," and yet she was willing to offer help. Her perceptive intuition and quick action provided us a quiet moment to breathe, relax, and receive a brief respite from our feisty boy. Her sacrifice of not worshiping with her husband that day was a priceless gift to a young couple in the throes of a whirling tornado. Her example has been one that I will never forget. Maybe because I am now a mother of three growing children who no longer require holding, bouncing, soothing, and constant consoling, I do know that if and when I see a young mother or young family in need of help, assistance, or aid, it is my *hope* and prayer that in that moment I will be willing to act with love and mercy, as the kind woman at church did for us.

Following his second birthday, Bennett's respiratory deficits were slowly improving but seizures continued to break through all medications we tried. It was torture to watch Bennett drool through a seizure as his left arm rhythmically pulsated. We were determined to find the best neurologist we could to get his seizures under control. Through word of mouth, we learned of a neurologist who had recently started his own practice and came highly recommended. Desperate for help, we booked an appointment with him and were anxious to get his opinion regarding the seizures. The relatively young neurologist read Bennett's complex medical history, listened to me as I explained my observations, and began brainstorming what he could do to help. He kept one of the seizure medications, added a new one, and after a few weeks with the new combination, Bennett's seizures were under control. Prior to this, I had begun to fear that we would never find a resolution to the seizures. Needless to say, we were cautiously optimistic.

In the fall of 2009 Travis accepted a job in Tennessee, so the commuting to D.C. stopped and we were grateful to spend our first official *Tender Tennessee Christmas* together with his family in December 2009. Travis got to know his new co-workers and we spent more time with his family and our friends. Our daily routines were reset to his new schedule, all while Bennett continued with his therapies and inclusive preschool. Life felt as if it was settling into a steady rhythm, but beneath the surface Travis was struggling. He tried to fake happiness, but eventually became unable to hide the pain. It was a struggle to get out of bed, and when he did, he was a pale and somber shell of his being.

In *The Body Keeps the Score* by Bessel van der Kolk, the author writes, "Our gut feelings signal what is safe, life-sustaining, or threatening, even if we cannot quite explain why we feel a particular way." Following Bennett's traumatic birth, Travis had worked tirelessly to provide for his family, care for Bennett, and support me. He cared for us flawlessly, and yet the trauma of Bennett's birth was a catalyst for so much that could no longer be ignored. Travis had gone through the motions methodically for nearly three years, and finally his body had reached its threshold for pain.

The flood

In May of 2010 Nashville experienced the now infamous "2010 Tennessee floods." These floods were considered "thousand-year floods" in Tennessee, Kentucky, and northern Mississippi, the result of torrential rains on May 1 and 2, 2010. Floods affected the area for several days afterwards as parts of downtown Nashville went underwater and even the Grand Ole Opry flooded. Tennessee recorded twenty-one deaths. Two-day rain totals in some areas were greater than nineteen inches. The Cumberland River crested at 51.86 feet in Nashville, a level not seen since 1937, which was before the US Army Corps of Engineers' flood-control measures were in place.

We watched our neighborhood go under water. Thankfully our ranch house was on higher ground, and we only experienced water in our crawl space. For days we monitored the weather reports as we watched the rain come pouring down. When breaks occurred amidst the endless rain, we pushed Bennett in his stroller along the streets of our neighborhood. We were shocked to observe rivers of water move through houses with rushing currents that swept furniture, décor, and debris downstream.

Bennett was two years old when those dark days of rain seemed to never end. We went about his daily routines, his giggles brought us great joy, but it was hard to break through in the darkness filling our house. The weight of Bennett's birth and diagnosis, depression creeping into our souls, disenchantment from Travis's new job, and a host of other feelings left us spinning in a pit of darkness. We consulted with the area's top mental health professionals, reached out to our faith community, and met with medical professionals who could help walk us through this bleak time—yet we had not addressed the trauma to us. The weight of it all left us feeling great despair and gloom. Gloom is the best word to describe the dark rolling clouds, the endless rain, the rushing rivers, the cries for help from people trapped in the water or houses literally destroyed in the darkness of the night. It was a tragic time for our beloved city, and it was an equally tragic time for the turmoil occurring inside our house. Words were at a minimum because the pain was so piercing that simply breathing encompassed all our energy. Getting out of bed was nearly impossible for us, but we knew there was a little boy depending on us for every need, so that responsibility helped to get us out of bed.

Eventually the sun came out after the flooding—the old cliché was true: the calm after the storm. Neighbors, churches, and strangers came to one another's aid as drywall was ripped out from houses completely ravaged by the rising water. Instead of waiting on government trucks to pull up to the city, the people of Nashville banded together and showed each other through their actions that they were going to literally "love thy neighbor as thyself." A flooded house is overwhelming and stressful. Time is of the essence to get it all dried out as soon as possible to avoid mold and toxins.

Numerous emails went around our social circles to see who needed help, so we mentioned to a friend that we were actually in need of a wet vacuum. Before we knew it, we had an acquaintance from our church show up with a wet vac to suck out all the water in our crawl space. It was a bright sunny day. He drove up to our house in his truck, simply got out of his truck, we spoke for a minute, he went around to our backyard, found the door to the crawlspace, and began working. I will never forget his act of kindness because there was no reason for this man to show up and help us. Throughout the state there were crises left and right. He had a wife and children at home, as well as a lot of family nearby. Yet he knew that we were a young family new to the area who had a son with severe disabilities, so he took the time out of his schedule to serve our family. Only the God of hope compels people to act this way!

> Thou shalt love the Lord thy God with thy whole heart, and with thy whole soul, and with thy whole mind. . . . And the second is like to this: Thou shalt love thy neighbor as thyself.
> — Matthew 22:37, 39

As the southeastern region of the United States recovered from the great flood, Travis and I had restoration coming for our hearts just over the horizon.

The four months that followed, from May through August 2010, included moments etched into our marriage of complete shock, devastation, and breakthrough. Travis reached out for help to several highly recommended professionals in the mental health space, the medical community, and the recovery community. In moments when he felt hopeless and desperate, there were people who cared about him enough to come sleep on our couch, bring us food, encourage him, or sit with us in our pain. Travis was surrounded by an army of people who refused to let him slip away into a world of isolation and anguish. I can say without a doubt that this army marched in line, linking arms with this weary man, carrying him through a very dark valley to the other side. Our army of support was willing to risk the journey because they deeply believed that Travis's life and our family were worth the arduous mental health journey that was before us.

On a sunny spring day in 2010 Travis was in a particularly unhealthy state of mind. His doctor called me to strongly advise that he be hospitalized immediately to be monitored for severe depression. Bennett and I drove him to the hospital, helped him register with a triage nurse, and watched him walk across the shiny beige linoleum tiles and disappear behind a large wooden door. Watching Travis walk away in such despair was heartbreaking, and yet it was a relief. I yearned for him to find peace and healing and knew that I could not be the one to give that to him. I drove home in tears, arrived home with Bennett, settled him in his crib, and noticed that I was feeling particularly tired and sick to my stomach. We had been open to having another child in early 2010, but had frankly forgotten about this possibility until it hit me like a ton of bricks. *Am I pregnant? No way. There is absolutely no way.*

Curious, I grabbed an extra pregnancy test from our medicine cabinet, and before I knew it I was holding a positive test result in my hand. In that moment, my fear could have gotten the best of me. *I had just checked my husband into the hospital.* I had a severely disabled child with a lifetime of needs ahead and a husband who was in the eye of a raging storm. I was working only part-time and hoped that Travis would be able to continue working, but if he needed time off to take care of his health, then I wanted him to do that. All I cared about was restoration, healing, and recovery for my husband who had carried the weight of our family for nearly three years. I held that test stick with its "plus" sign, I smiled, I cried, and was covered in total peace. A peace that passes all understanding.

A few days later, Travis phoned and told me he was being discharged. I was relieved to hear his voice and could not wait to see him. I arranged to leave Bennett with Travis's mother while I pondered whether to tell Travis the exciting news I had just found out. I did not want to add any stress or anxiety to his heart and mind, and yet I knew how much he longed for more children. I felt in my core that this good news might lift him up. Seeing Travis's bright blue eyes, as he walked out to our car in the circle drive and hopped in, took my breath away. He looked good. He looked more peaceful. He looked as if he had eaten, and was no longer an emaciated pale zombie.

We drove to one of our favorite parks south of Nashville, not far from our house, and we sat on the hill overlooking the mountain range, green grass, and houses sprinkled throughout the countryside. The cool spring breeze danced across our faces, and I knew in my heart that I must tell him. It was not my news. It was our news. I had no idea how far along I was, but regardless, this was his child growing inside of me and Travis deserved to be made aware of it.

We small-talked for a few minutes, and then I blurted, "Well, I have some good news and some bad news. Which would you like first?" He said he didn't care, so I replied, "The bad news is that I really have not felt well these past few days. The good news is that it is because I am pregnant." His eyes lit up brightly and glimmered the way they do when his smile beams. "You have no idea how happy this makes me, babe." Any anxiety that I had over the decision to tell him was washed away as we hugged, cried, and took a moment to soak in the hope of this new gift. Bennett was going to be a big brother.

My nausea was relentless, and I craved protein nonstop. Not just hard-boiled eggs, bacon, or cheese, but a super-sized Arby's double roast beef sandwich, something I had never before in my life eaten. My clothes got tight quickly, and we decided to tell our parents in the first trimester after seeing a strong heartbeat at our first ultrasound. I knew that my mom probably thought I had been acting "off" and not like my normal self, so I was bustling with excitement to share with her our wonderful news.

We soon gathered my mom and Travis's parents around our lunch table one bright and sunny spring day. The sun's rays shone through our sliding glass door as we watched their responses while they unfolded a printed copy of the ultrasound announcing, "Speck Baby #2 coming soon," which had been folded into large Easter eggs placed on each of their plates.

Travis's parents carefully unfolded their ultrasound picture, smiled, cheered, and gave us hugs while my mom sat quietly in her chair with tears rolling down her cheeks. She had been the one person to see up close and personal many of our challenges raising Bennett and she was frankly terrified. I was taken aback by her tears of what looked like sadness, but she quickly clarified that she was only scared, very scared. We hugged, reassured her that everything was looking great, and she eventually laughed and smiled, declaring, "When I saw you wearing that horrible brown mousy dress I knew that something was up. I thought to myself, 'That does not look like something Kelly would wear!'"

My pregnancy was a time of delight and dreams, and yet it was a time of more roller coasters. I was followed by an obstetrician and considered high-risk because of the way that Bennett's pregnancy had ended. Our obstetrician (OB) was doing frequent ultrasounds to watch the baby's growth, and all signs were looking great. Following Travis's initial hospitalization, we followed his care plan diligently, so some weeks he seemed well-supported and on the path to full restoration. Other weeks it seemed as if nothing was working to ease his deep pain, and the job he had taken in Nashville had turned out to be a toxic wasp nest.

It became clear that we needed more support, so Travis agreed to enroll in a twenty-eight-day program for intensive individual and group support. His brother and I drove him there, gave him huge hugs, and then he walked behind a closed door. The registration gentleman looked me in the eyes and said, "Ma'am, your husband is on the verge of a nervous breakdown. He seems like a really great guy and I sincerely mean that. I think the guy just needs a break." Travis did need a break. It had all turned out to be just too much. Watching his son nearly bleed to death. Working all day in a stressful environment, then coming home to hear a baby screaming for hours. Moving in with his mother-in-law for a year. Moving his family to another state while commuting each week by plane. Realizing his new job was a bad decision. It was just too much.

Travis completed the program and came home rested, restored, and renewed. He soon thereafter resigned from his toxic job and began an expansive search for another job in Nashville. He looked around for any job he was remotely qualified for, but there were no fits compatible with his experience. We were living off our savings, were paying large health insurance premiums, and both felt the pressure rising while the clock was ticking toward the arrival of our second son. One hot and humid July day, while Travis was working in the flower bed in our backyard, he came into the house and told me, "We need to go back to D.C. I think the Lord just told me we need to go back to D.C., while I was outside shoveling mulch." I was both shocked and relieved because

I had actually been thinking the very same thing. I loved Tennessee and our home there had been a shelter for healing, yet there was something deep within my heart that was nudging me to be open to the option to move back.

Travis made one phone call to his previous boss. His boss was about to post a position, and Travis was offered the position with a start date that allowed us to move and get settled before the birth of our second child. God showed up for us once again: this time not during a life-or-death crisis, but rather the agonizing process of a bleak job search, a growing baby in my womb, and a two-and-a-half-year-old with medical needs that were specific and not cheap. The details were ironed out by God's providing a renter for our Tennessee house, a rental in Bethesda, Maryland, and a wonderful job opportunity. We had no choice but to jump at the chance. All the signs were showing that the Tennessee chapter of our lives was closing. It was time to move north, settle in, find a school for Bennett, and have a baby. And have a baby we soon did.

On November 2, 2010, we welcomed Jackson Stafford Speck to this world with great relief and happiness. We were head over heels in love with him from the moment we saw his chubby little cheeks. Jackson's birth brought healing, peace, and joy to crevasses in our hearts that we did not fully know even existed. His planned C-section was flawless, and he came out bright red, screaming his head off. His deep blue eyes melted us from day one. He was a serious little guy who would stare us down in our hospital room as we changed his diaper or held him close. Jackson was also a sensitive child from the minute he was born. He continues to be that way to this day. The birth of Jackson, a pink, squishy, stout and healthy son, soothed the lingering pain of Bennett's traumatic birth experience and restored us in significant ways.

As Jackson grows, we are blown away by God's wisdom in giving us exactly the second son that we needed. Before Jackson was even a year old, if we handed him a ball, he would bat it around like a Harlem Globetrotter. He was scooting around our hardwood floors, lodging himself under furniture, and soon crawling like lightning throughout our house at alarmingly early ages. Jackson's agility was off the charts, yet he has always been a cuddly snuggler, particularly at night. There were many nights in his early years of life when I walked past his room to see Travis sitting in the glider there, rocking back and forth, holding Jackson asleep on his shoulder. Both their eyes would be closed, their chests breathing together in peaceful harmony. The sight took my breath away. These simple gifts of normalcy brought renewal to our hearts in profound ways.

CHAPTER 14

Great Pain (Travis's Story)

"When God wants to do an impossible task,
He takes an impossible man and crushes him."
— Alan Redpath

S HOCK, DISMAY, and total fear ran through my veins in greater supply than blood. All I wanted was to be with Bennett and Kelly, but I was with neither of them just a few moments after Kelly gave birth. While Bennett was lying in the small NICU bay at Sibley Memorial Hospital in D.C., I sat in a swivel chair in a back office not far away asking the attending physician what we were looking at in a worst-case scenario. I guess it is just my personality, but I wanted the truth and I wanted it now, regardless of how bad the outcome may be. *How bad could this be anyway, right? We are in the hospital in the nation's capital with world-class medical care all around us. Whatever this is, it will be okay. Cut to the chase, please.* I was unprepared for what the doctor told me next. But before she even said a word, her eyes alone told my gut that this was more serious than I even understood at that moment. Looking at me in strength but with great compassion, she said, "Mr. Speck, the worst-case scenario is that Bennett will have cerebral palsy." And with those thirteen brief words, our lives changed forever.

Kelly has already mentioned that we both used to be very Type-A personalities, planning and controlling our way through life. We are both recovering control addicts. We all have this tendency to some degree, because it is simply human nature. But our long and tragic NICU experience had a way of opening the blinds and shedding full light on just how much of an issue this was in our lives. No project plan prepares you for this. No series of better or different choices prepares you for this. No guidance, training, or advice prepares you for this. One day you are walking along in seemingly full control of your life and future, and the next minute you are pushed off of a cliff and wondering how in the world the free fall started, and why.

But the free fall had indeed started, and for me personally, an unanticipated consequence was the gradual but persistent death of my old self beginning that August morning of Bennett's birth. You see, up until that point in my life, I had been a perfectionist. I was a stoic. I was a stoic perfectionist who actually took great pride in both approaches—after all, they had worked quite well for me. But there is nothing in this world that cuts you like the sight of your child, your firstborn child at that, covered and soaked in blood and suffering in front of you. It was a quick and sudden blow to the core of who I was, and the protection that stoicism had provided for me all my life received its first death blow.

But the death blows continued. A few years prior to Bennett's birth, I had begun experiencing severe migraine headaches. They were terrible. A well-known neurologist in town prescribed strong narcotic pain medications for the headaches, but for the first few years I would never even take those medications. I did not feel that my level of migraine pain had warranted the heavy-hitter narcotics. After Bennett's birth experience and the emotional toll it took on me, that very medication became the best way I knew how to cope with that level of physical and emotional pain. The headaches continued, but so did the use and eventually the abuse of the medication, more for emotional than physically-related purposes. I thought a move home to my beloved state of Tennessee would do the trick and help me cope with my new reality of raising a severely disabled child, yet the abuse of the medication worsened. Eventually it exploded into clinical depression, terrible anxiety, and full-blown panic attacks that made me wish I were dead. It finally culminated in a hospitalization and a month-long stay at a rehabilitation facility. The reliance on myself had finally been brought to its knees and forced to unconditionally surrender.

Prior to Bennett's birth, and as embarrassing as it is to say this, there were three groups of people I never much empathized with or even desired to be around: people who complained about migraine headaches (*just take a Tylenol, for crying out loud, and stop whining!*); families who have children with severe disabilities; and those suffering from mental illness and addiction. It's amazing what deep and identity-altering suffering does for one's perspective and priorities in life. Only suffering can produce the results it produces. Today, my love, admiration, and respect for these three groups of heavenly people could not be higher. I consider this one of the blessings or "fruits" of the suffering since that fateful day in August of 2007 for which I remain grateful. It could not have happened any other way.

The Lord takes away, but the Lord also gives, and He is a God of restoration. When Bennett was born, he could not have been sicker. When Jackson was born, he could not have been healthier. I would never be able to converse with my firstborn son, but my second-born was stronger than an ox. To this day, he rarely even gets sick with a cold. He is literally one of the strongest kids I have ever known. I knew early on that with Jackson, my experience as a father to a son would finally take on a more typical pattern, and there is not a day that goes by that I am not deeply grateful for that. He is very special to me, and I am extremely proud to be his daddy. Spending time with him in any way is one of the things I most treasure and what makes me the happiest today.

And the giving and restoration continued. Our third-born, Reagan Jean, was born a little less than two years after Jackson, and Daddy finally had his little girl. Reagan looks just like me, while Jackson looks just like Kelly. It is really quite amazing. But Reagan is definitely her father's daughter, and the love and laughter that she has brought to our family is impossible to quantify. As Kelly later reveals, Reagan was actually born with a birth defect. While this was initially very difficult news to accept and process, and it has been painful to watch her experience numerous doctor appointments and surgeries (with more on the way), walking the path with Reagan has been easier for us to face in comparison to the trauma of Bennett's birth experience. Reagan, like her mother, is absolutely gorgeous on the outside and inside. I am blessed to have such a beautiful and loving daughter, and I treasure the unique gifts the Lord has given her.

Without question, the only reason that Kelly and I stand today and share our experience with you is because of our faith in God, and in His mighty and only Son, Jesus Christ. When word first spread of Bennett's condition, a good friend of mine sent me a text that simply said the following: "Be strong, mighty man of God." I've never really considered myself a mighty man of anything, but there is no question that my primary identity had already been deeply forged in my life up until that point as a follower of God. This identity was forged from a lifetime of influence from family, friends, and experiences that formed the foundation for the fortress that would be needed to weather the storm Kelly and I now found ourselves facing. The text was a reminder to me very early on that no matter what we faced in the days and years ahead, we could do it because of the unique power that was with and in us in that Name.

The cornerstone of that foundation is love. Not long after bringing Bennett home from the hospital, I found myself speaking about the experience at our church in Fairfax as we celebrated communion together. Our church had been a huge source of strength and support during Bennett's stay in the NICU. I remarked that up until that point I had always only distantly related to God's experience of watching His only Son suffer and bleed to death on a cross. I now found myself much more closely and emotionally involved in the divine moment that changed the course of history and eternity unlike any before or since. Yet I could not help but notice a big difference in my experience and God's.

You see, as I looked down and watched Bennett's immense suffering, bleeding, and torturous pain in his NICU bay, had I had any power at that time to end it I would have stopped it all immediately and without hesitation. That is probably no surprise to you. But God, who has all power and dominion and authority, when he looked down at His own Son suffering, bleeding, and in torturous pain on the cross at Calvary, allowed it to continue right in front of Him. It is one kind of love to want the pain and suffering of your child to end but not have the power to change it, but it's another kind of love altogether to watch your child suffer, have power to end it all, and yet allow it to continue and finish in the child's death. That kind of love, when fully understood and grasped, does not just change the way you think; it changes the way you live. It changes everything about you. It is not possible to come into full contact with that kind of love and not be changed forever.

Even so—and let me be clear and very transparent about this—it has not been easy, and there have been many struggles that continue to this day. Things can be extremely difficult when raising a family that includes a precious child with severe disabilities. Many questions, uncertainties, fears, and struggles remain, and these often stalk us throughout our days and weeks. Emotions are pressed hard and run thin, and often they spill over. We are definitely not perfect in any way, and we make mistakes very often. We grow fearful of the future, we have unanswered questions, and ongoing challenges make us often wonder how we are going to do this. We do not always have answers and remain uncertain of many things.

But we are also more certain than ever of the things that matter more than anything else. We have been blessed with wonderful parents, family, and friends who have given so much to sustain and encourage us on this journey; it would take another whole book to list them and spell out all the ways they have helped us. One family mentor in particular, Bob Scott, who has since passed away, told me and Kelly many things in the cherished times we met with him and his precious wife Bernice during our college years in Abilene in the great state of Texas. They lovingly "adopted" college "grandkids," offering them hot meals and a place to stay whenever needed. On certain Sundays, Bernice would prepare a delicious home-cooked meal (usually melt-in-your-mouth Texas barbeque brisket) while Bob would spur conversation with those college kids sitting around their dining room table. Bob told us things that we remember constantly in our day-to-day lives; things like, "There are no unimportant people in this life" and "All people are created in the image of God, and therefore have great dignity, value, and worth."

He told Kelly and me many other things like this that we treasure to this day and are grateful for. Yet without question my favorite one that he would tell us regularly, and the one which has enabled us to hope when all hope seemed lost, was that "God will never leave you or forsake you. He will always be with you wherever you go." In our last visit with Bob, he looked at Kelly and me and simply said, "May the Lord bless you and be with you *momento* by *momento*."

That is what we are most confident of today and what gives us our source of hope—that His Presence will be with us and sustain us each minute, hour, and day of the year. That is what I know. He was there through it all, and He still is, providing for and sustaining us day by day, moment by moment. People have sometimes looked at us and wondered how or why we would choose to still hope, to still love and follow a God that would allow all that has happened to Bennett, allowed our individual struggles, and the stress placed on our marriage. Our response to this is simply the same as the ancient words of Peter when he looked at Jesus and said, "To whom then shall we go?" (John 6:68).

The source of the hope determines the quality of the hope. One day, when eternity finally comes, I know that I will finally hear Bennett say the word that I have longed to hear from him since the moment he was born: "Daddy." This moment will happen, I am sure of it. It will happen because of the hope and peace that only God can provide.

Hope humbly then; with trembling pinions soar;
Wait the great teacher Death; and God adore!
What future bliss, He gives not thee to know,
But gives that hope to be thy blessing now.
Hope springs eternal in the human breast:
Man never is, but always to be blest:
The soul, uneasy and confin'd from home,
Rests and expatiates in a life to come.
— Alexander Pope

CHAPTER 15

Bennett is a Big Brother and Starts School

"I believe that education is all about being excited about something."
— Steve Irwin

HAVING TWO SONS as our first children was a time of great joy for us. Bennett was a happy three-year-old preschooler, and Jackson was a strong and observant infant who studied our every move. When Jackson entered the world, he stared us down from the start. He has always been a hard kid to win over. We had to work hard for every smile or giggle, but after he trusted us and knew he could count on us, he handed out those smiles and giggles with abundance. He is still a hard nut to crack. He is intense, sensitive, and laser focused on whatever he is doing.

Soon after Jackson was born, he was always hungry (unfortunately my milk supply was not enough), so he screamed his head off after nursing until we "topped him off" with a formula bottle. He then lazily looked up at us, milk-drunk, and stared at us as if to say, "Next time please have the bottle set and ready. I do not like having to wait."

Changing Jackson's diaper was like wrestling a wet seal, and his well-visit checkups usually entailed the pediatrician noting his fierce leg strength and ability to dodge the vaccination needles. Jackson's maternal grandmother felt constantly rejected by the fact that he did not want a thing to do with her until he was a preschooler, even as she came bearing gifts with each visit. The child has always been strong-willed, and he simply cannot fake what he does not feel. I admire this particularly authentic trait of his.

A week after Jackson was born, Bennett was scheduled to begin a special-needs preschool as a three-year-old in our local public-school system. Apparently, I had agreed to have the bus pick him up in front of our rental house and drive him seven miles to the school. In the fog of my sleep-deprived existence, when the day of Bennett's first day of preschool arrived, I was close to a full-on panic attack. Thoughts were darting through my head as I got him dressed and ready for his big day: *How can I kiss his cheeks, place my toddler in his stroller (a.k.a. supportive small wheelchair), wheel him onto his short yellow bus's chair lift, and wave goodbye as a stranger drives off with him? By the way, this stranger is driving my baby on the interstate Beltway that wraps around Washington, D.C. Why did I ever think this was a good idea?*

So here is what happened. I greeted the kind bus driver who looked like Bob Marley's long-lost twin, pushed Bennett onto the chairlift, and watched his chair slowly elevate up onto the bus. I then watched the attendant secure his wheelchair straps and buckle Bennett's chair in place. I immediately took Jackson's infant carrier straight to the car, hopped into the driver's seat while my mom hopped into the passenger seat, and we followed the bus every single mile to the school.

We quickly pulled into a parking spot at his school, got out of the car, and watched as our little miracle boy was wheeled into his school for the very first time. The tears flowed down our cheeks as we took a moment to feel the weight of this momentous event. The educational journey of Bennett Mitchell Speck began in November 2010 at a local school that had been serving children with "profound and severe" disabilities in our county for nearly fifty years. The building had sheltered thousands of little saints, many of whom had stayed from preschool at age three to graduation at age twenty-one, per the Individuals with Disabilities Education Act (IDEA):

The Individuals with Disabilities Education Act (IDEA) is a law that makes available a free appropriate public education to eligible children with disabilities throughout the nation and ensures special education and related services to those children.

The IDEA governs how states and public agencies provide early intervention, special education, and related services to more than 7.5 million (as of school year 2018-19) eligible infants, toddlers, children, and youth with disabilities.

Infants and toddlers, birth through age two, with disabilities and their families receive early intervention services under IDEA Part C. Children and youth ages three through 21 receive special education and related services under IDEA Part B.

Sending Bennett to our public-school system began a journey of introductions to incredible educators, staff, and therapists. He had the opportunity to attend his school from age three to age twenty-one. During the first spring of his preschool year, a small group of parents organized a "Spring Fling" event where there was a moon-bounce, snacks, games, and fundraising on a hot, sticky, Maryland day in May. We eagerly attended as a family of four, the boys wearing orange-and-blue-striped matching shirts. Our excitement about meeting other families and teachers was palpable. This was our new community and we were glad to get involved.

As we walked up to a small group of parents, two moms came forward and welcomed us to the school community. We made small talk for a few moments. I learned that the children of these moms were teenagers and had been educated in there for several years. I shared that we were new parents at S.K.S., and one mother said "Welcome! It's a wild ride! I mean, never in my life could I imagine I would be changing my twelve-year-old son's diapers." Caught off guard by her alarming comment, I pushed out a nervous laugh, chatted for a bit more, thanked them for planning the day, and we proceeded to make our way to the colorful moon bounce. I appreciated the mom's honesty, and yet it felt as if I had been punched in the stomach. I had not exactly looked ahead to what Bennett would be like at the age of twelve, nor could I imagine the level of caretaking that we would be doing then. We had entered a whole new world. Our hope was green.

Once we arrived at the moon bounce, we realized it was full of kids and our two sons were actually too small to participate, and the heat and humidity were sweltering. We were all covered in sweat, the boys were ready for fluids and a nap, and their parents needed some time to process this new world we had stepped into. Travis and I were grateful to have met several parents who understood our life. They too had kids who were not "typical" or "normal" in their development, and yet they were devoted to their children with a deep love that is hard to put into mere words. The Spring Fling day back in 2011 was a good and sobering day for our family. This new world was beautiful, jarring, unconventional, and unexpected.

Through the years at Bennett's incredible school, he has had some truly gifted teachers, deeply caring para-educators, amazing therapists, and passionate administrators who are committed to building the best educational experience available for children with disabilities, like Bennett. We have been involved in the small parent-leadership group, we have planned staff appreciation breakfasts, attended school-sponsored family events, and done our best to show our support and appreciation for the important work that is done at this school.

One especially sweet gift that came from Bennett's school is a special person named Arlene. Bennett first met Arlene while he was in preschool, and their friendship took off from there. Arlene's joyous smile, soothing voice, and fantastic laugh brought an electric energy to the halls of the school. One day at pickup she told me, "Mrs. Speck, did you know that Benny loves Elton John? I sing "Benny and the Jets" to him all day long and he busts out laughing every time. He loves that song!" We had no idea this had become Bennett's anthem at school with Ms. Arlene, so it immediately became a song we sang to him at home as well. To this day Bennett lights up with a big grin whenever we start singing Elton John's song. Arlene moved schools and is no longer with Bennett, but she still comes over to our house regularly to visit, sit with Bennett, or help us out by caring for him when we have events outside the home that he would not enjoy. Bennett loves staying at home with Arlene to listen in on her conversations. He loves the sound of her soulful voice, and as she always says, "Benny, you are so nosy listening in on all my conversations; that's always what you do at school is listen in on the adult chatter!"

I had the privilege of speaking at two of Bennett's school graduations, cheering extra loudly for the kids who were "lifers" after attending from age three to age twenty-one. As I looked at graduates with deep respect for them and their families, I hoped with all my heart (amidst my tears) that one day Bennett would be graduating as well. The reality at our school is that every year that we have been there, a white envelope with the school's return address shows up in our mailbox. Most times, I grab the envelope with the rest of our mail, it gets plopped on our kitchen counter, and when the envelope is eventually opened I am shaken by the words from the principal announcing the sudden passing of one of Bennett's peers. Some years there have been announcements of more than one student perishing, and it guts me to my core. Each time I typically stand stunned as I read the words, I cry and I pray for the family experiencing the great loss, and for our family, who might one day have to embrace this devastating loss ourselves.

Medically fragile children, children with "severe and profound" disabilities, or "non-typical" developing children all exist with such great challenges and physical and/or genetic complexities that each moment they are alive is a miracle. For example, for kids with seizure disorders, for each day that their little brains function without a seizure (or a "glitch," as my two video-game-loving kids like to call seizures), parents like us sigh a deep breath of relief and press on to face the next day of unknowns. Because we have been experiencing this "life of unknowns" since the day Bennett was born, we feel oddly at home when at Bennett's school, surrounded by parents who understand our reality.

When Bennett's preschool graduation was being planned in the spring of 2012 by his superb teacher, Ms. Yvonne, she mentioned to me that in years past sometimes a parent would say a few words. At this point I had Bennett, age four, Jackson, age one, and was very pregnant and swollen with Reagan. I was in no condition to speak before a group of parents, staff, and students, but I did have a handsome husband who could sing. I went home, asked Travis if he would be comfortable singing a song for Bennett's preschool graduation, and after some extended convincing, he agreed to sing the inspiring song "The River" by Garth Brooks. When the day of Bennett's preschool graduation finally arrived, the school gym was filled with our beloved teachers and staff, nervous parents, fidgety preschoolers, and Bennett in his wheelchair wearing his cap and gown. "Pomp and Circumstance" blared from the loudspeakers, and Bennett was rolled into his spot where he sat and then listened to his daddy sing to him and his classmates, "Lord, I will sail my vessel 'til the river runs dry." Bennett kicked with glee throughout.

As we walk together along the roller coaster life of Individualized Education Plans (IEPs), meetings, and esting required for special education, Travis and I hold tight to the hope that Bennett will be happy and continue to thrive as he inches toward that final momentous graduation day at the age of twenty. (He will turn twenty-one right before the next school year begins and therefore would not be eligible to enroll that year.) It is our hope that one day we will dress him in his best outfit, and he will proudly wear his red cap and gown as he is wheeled down the middle aisle, surrounded by friends and family cheering him on. As we watch him with tears rolling down our faces, "Pomp and Circumstance" will be playing over the loudspeaker located between the bright green ferns. What a day of celebration we hope and pray that will be.

Our blue-eyed surprise

"Life is tough, my darling, but so are you." — *Stephanie Bennet Henry*
Toward the end of December 2011 when Bennett was four and Jackson was one, I had a sour stomach that would not go away. No matter what I ate, the dull nausea would not lift. I tried everything from Tums to crackers to chicken broth. We had made plans to travel with the boys to visit Travis's family in Tennessee, and on the drive down a thought jolted into my mind. Am I pregnant? As I thought more about it, this sour-stomach feeling did remind me of the early days of pregnancy with Bennett and Jackson. Oh my. Surely not. As I did a few calculations in my head, I did not think this was really possible.

Before pulling onto Travis's parents' street, I asked him to stop at a local pharmacy store so I could run in to quickly "buy some gum." I bought a pregnancy test, along with some gum, and popped back into the car to see my three handsome fellas smiling back at me. Jackson had just turned one year old a month prior to this, so as I looked at his chubby cheeks, bright blue eyes, and toothy grin, I wondered to myself, "Is he going to be a big brother?"

A few hours later that question was answered. Indeed, both Jackson and Bennett were going to be big brothers. We once again confirmed via a clear vertical line on a plastic stick indicating we were "pregnant." We later sat around the oval wooden kitchen table covered in a red checkered tablecloth with Travis's parents, sister, and her family, where Travis proudly announced that next Christmas Grana would have seven grandchildren (one more than the six she had at that time). They all jumped for joy, we grinned, and the celebration of a new life was the best Christmas gift we could have ever imagined that December in 2011.

The nausea continued with my third pregnancy, as it had with my first two. Most days I was able to keep my stomach calm with carbs and the distractions of caring for the boys and working part-time. We had not told many people we were pregnant, apart from family, as we assumed most folks would think we had lost our minds for having a third child, considering our atypical circumstances and the fact that the boys were only four and one at the time.

We wanted to find out what our third baby's sex was, so when the big twenty-week appointment approached on our calendar, our hearts were thrilled. Either way, we were excited about this baby. We honestly felt that three boys would be delightful, or news of a baby girl would simply be perfect. Anyone who has sat in an ultrasound room with belly exposed and cold jelly-like substance rubbed onto it to guide the ultrasound wand might agree that the experience is intense yet peaceful.

The two boys were with a babysitter, so Travis and I were alone in the ultrasound room that gray and gloomy April day. The ultrasound tech asked us if we were finding out the sex of the baby, we said yes, and she then told us it was time for me to go shopping for our baby girl. We were surprised, having both assumed it was going to be Boy Number Three. We were thrilled and then sucker-punched when the tech's face tensed, the air in the room got still, and she quickly said, "I will be right back."

As I lay on the table making small talk with Travis about our baby-girl news, my gut was hoping that the tech was simply using the restroom, but deep in my soul I knew that there was bad news coming. Moments prior to this I had read her face and body language and knew that something was off. After what felt like an hour passed, the ultrasound tech re-entered the room and said that a doctor would be in shortly to talk to us regarding something that they had seen on the monitor. A kind female OB then entered the room, smiled, and shared with us that our baby girl appeared to have a cleft lip, a common birth defect that can be fixed by surgery once she was born. The images were not clear enough to show if the baby's palate would be intact, and they could not see the four chambers of her heart to know if there were any heart defects, so she recommended that we schedule an ultrasound at Children's National Hospital as soon as possible. She asked us if we had any more questions, we said no, and we were then left alone in the room to make sense of this news.

Flabbergasted is not a strong enough word to encapsulate our feelings as we sat alone in the dark, cold hospital room that day. After all we had been through with Bennett, we had naïvely assumed that we had "suffered enough" and could rely on the fact that "God would not give us more than we could handle." Frankly, in that moment, this situation felt like more than we could handle. The OB told us that she did not think that the baby had a heart defect, but explained that cleft lips can be related to heart defects, so the heaviness of the possibility weighed on us like a sopping wet towel. We later learned that one in seven hundred babies are born with a cleft lip around the world (0.14 percent of all births). Of those babies with clefts, 24 percent will have a cleft lip on its own and 31 percent will have a cleft lip and palate. We did not know whether we would be falling within the 24 or 31 percent groups. Lucky us. We were once again dealing with being an anomaly and it was devastating.

We drove away from the hospital that day deflated and disillusioned. The sky was gray, a wet chill was in the air, and a silence filled our van. I did not have a pep talk cued up in my back pocket to give Travis, for I had not prepared myself for anything but "normal" and "good" news from our ultrasound for our third child. As I dropped Travis back off at his office building, I recall mumbling something like, "Everything is going to be okay. We have to trust that." Travis nodded, gave me a kiss on the cheek, and quietly left the car. My heart ached as I watched him walk along the path and through the security gate into his office building. My husband was clearly distraught, and I was stunned. Once again, I felt punched in my gut.

For the next twenty weeks I was in a swirl of fog and somehow cared for Bennett while chasing an active one-year-old who could run faster than his puffy, pregnant mother. I had no words. I trusted God, and yet I was baffled and afraid. As a result, I could pray only three words: "I trust You." God knew every meditation of my heart, all my thoughts and feelings, and yet through my disillusionment all I could physically muster from my lips were the words "I trust You." And I did. He had performed miracles and been with us every step of the way since Bennett's birth. I knew He would not abandon us now, so I clung tightly to a Bible verse that had been recited to me many times:

"Trust in the Lord with all your heart and lean not on your own understanding. In all your ways acknowledge Him, and He shall make your paths straight." — Proverbs 3:5-6

I had numerous ultrasounds throughout the second half of my pregnancy, and they all gave us encouraging news. Her heart presented as healthy, all other organs were exactly where they were supposed to be, and yet they could never get a clear view of her palate, so we had to simply wait and see what we had when she was delivered. In this age of modern medicine, it was hard to accept the fact that her palate structure was unknown based on the high-contrast ultrasounds, but we heeded the professionals' findings and continued with our prayer of "I trust You."

For anyone who knows our daughter, you will not be surprised to know that we had scheduled her C-section but she decided to pick her own arrival date. Attempting to stay cool on another thick humid night, we ran to a local frozen-yogurt shop after dinner on August 14. I could barely walk due to shooting sciatic-nerve pain running down the backs of my legs, so we each got our favorite flavors and toppings and ate our frozen yogurt in the car with the boys happily strapped into their car seats. Travis and I sat there downing the cold smooth treats, attempting to muster the energy to go home and put the boys to sleep for the night. Once the boys were tucked into bed, Travis quickly crashed onto our bed, I went to shower, and as I stood in the old iron shower of our 1951 Cape Cod home, I felt a gush of water break. My water had broken.

The baby had decided she wanted out, and therefore we needed to get to the hospital as soon as possible. After our journey with Bennett, we had plenty of trauma surrounding the words "bacteria" or "infection," so the last thing we wanted was any additional complications. I was nervous that my contractions might start ramping up soon, so I waddled into our room, shook Travis from his deep sleep, and told him my water had just broken. "You have got to be kidding," he replied. I wished that I were kidding, but nope. It was game time.

Quickly I called my mom who lived about forty minutes away, waking her, and asked her to come stay at our house overnight with the two boys. In a state of worried shock, she agreed and threw a few personal items into a bag before jumping into her car. There was no traffic at that time of night. Normally the trip could have taken up to an hour and a half, but she was able to race around the Beltway and across the eight-lane bridge over the Potomac River to Maryland in no time.

We also called Travis's mother in Tennessee, who already had a flight booked on the day of the scheduled C-section and asked her to change it and come the next day. It was going to take a village to care for our family including Bennett, age four, Jackson, age twenty months, and a newborn baby girl with a lot of unknowns. Not to mention I was having my third C-section and would not be able to lift anything heavier than a gallon of milk. We gathered our team, necessary to survive the coming weeks.

Travis and I arrived at the Georgetown Hospital Emergency Room entrance where they quickly admitted me, put me in a wheelchair, and Travis wheeled me up to Labor and Delivery. They asked me when my last food intake was, I mentioned the frozen yogurt, and they said we would have to wait eight hours after food intake before they could perform the C-section. By this point it was about midnight, so I calculated that we would be heading into the operating room at four o'clock in the morning, at the earliest.

I looked over at Travis's drooping eyelids and bloodshot eyes, and immediately knew it would be a long, exhausting night. He attempted to sleep in an upright chair while sitting next to me, and I tried to close my eyes here and there as they monitored both me and the baby all night long. The fetal monitors all showed that the baby was looking "happy" and contractions did not really ever get going, or, if they did, my eventual epidural helped block all of that pain. We were quite sure this was going to be our last baby, so I tried to breathe deeply and take in the entire experience, while pushing down any fear or dread that crept into my heart about what we might encounter after the doctors pulled her from my womb. There were many unknowns surrounding her birth, and yet my deepest gut feeling kept assuring me that everything would be fine.

The nurses and doctors prepared for surgery in the wee hours of the morning on August 15, 2012, and before we knew it, Reagan Jean Speck was born at a healthy seven pounds, five ounces. The kind female OB pulled her out, cleaned her off, brought Reagan around to see us and said, "Mom and Dad, you have a beautiful and healthy baby girl. Her palate is fully intact." Reagan's eyes locked with mine, I caught a glimpse of her sparkle, and an instant peace immediately washed over me. Her cleft lip was flipped out and her left nostril was deformed, yet those huge blue eyes stared into my soul, and I knew that my best girl had finally arrived. She was strong, she was mighty, and that twinkle in her eye told me she was all set to begin this life with us, her crazy family.

CHAPTER 16
Losses

*"I'm unsure which pain is worse—the shock of
what happened or the ache for what never will."*
— Author Unknown

ONE SPRING MORNING in 2011 we picked up bagels for breakfast at a local deli, and took a family walk with the two boys strapped into our double jogging stroller. The boys were ages four and one. As we strolled up to a local park where a T-ball game was happening, Travis stopped, stared dazedly through the chain-link fence, and the look on his face crushed my heart. I could almost see into his mind. *Bennett should be out on that field learning how to swing a bat.*

Travis likely would have been his first coach, cheering him on as he ran the bases and sprinted toward home plate, arms flailing. We gazed down at Bennett who was strapped in securely, unable to sit up independently, let alone run. The fact that he was alive to push in a stroller was in itself a miracle. And yet hand-in-hand with this miracle are stinging losses along the way, and the stings are continuous. With each "typical" milestone that happens in life, the stings are real. Some stings throb more than others.

We have tried hard to name those losses and feelings of sadness or despair when the waves either hit us in the face (or sneakily creep into the crevasses of our hearts). The more we push those hard feelings down, pressing them back to the far corners of our hearts and minds, the more feelings come back with a vengeance in times of frustration, loneliness, or overwhelmed emotions.

It reminds me of a particularly hard night in the NICU back when Bennett was two months old and had just had the MRI revealing his brain damage and diagnosis. We were wrestling with the news and our dear nurse Adele could tell that we were having a hard time processing all that Bennett's cerebral palsy diagnosis meant for our lives. *Would he ever walk? Would he ever talk? Would he be able to play sports?*

"Bennett is exactly the child God intended him to be," Adele told us gently as her deep brown eyes stared directly into ours. Her statement was so simple and yet so profound. Some people may have brushed it off or come up with a secular rebuttal. But her words hung in the air like honey as we both nodded in agreement. I will never forget the sentence that Adele spoke over us. Her words were given as a charge to us, and we have referred back to that statement multiple times throughout Bennett's life.

There truly have been many ironies in our parenting journey, and the journey is far from over. Our first child could not initially breathe, eat by mouth, or bring his hands together to hold a bottle. He spent months of his early life agitated and screaming, and growth and weight gain have always been a struggle. As a result, we learned to take nothing for granted. Our second child ate anything we offered him, was agile from the moment he started jumping in his crib at seven months old, and was noted by the pediatrician as an "alpha male" at his one-year well-visit appointment. He is sensitive (like his mom), and has always been the child who needs the reassuring security, connection, and routine. Our baby girl had a wide gap in her mouth/nasal area that perfectly latched onto whichever nipple was given to her, contributing to off-the-charts growth. Every well-visit check-in has concluded her growth is above 99 percent of normal. She is her daddy's twin as she has the strength of a lion and a heart of gold. Our three children literally could not be more different. They do not look like siblings; they share very few, if any, attributes; and yet they somehow came from the same DNA of their two biological parents. Yet in the early days when all three were in diapers, each weighing about the same, it nearly felt like we were raising triplets. Each child had incredibly unique needs—both medically and emotionally—and many days we did not know if we were capable of individually meeting the needs set before us. We wondered how we would survive (and keep them all alive) as toddler Jackson pulled over a lamp onto himself and Bennett, or when Reagan tumbled down the carpeted stairs as we were busy amidst bedtime routines. Placing all three of them in the bathtub together was the only assurance that all parties were present and accounted for.

Jackson and Reagan's development quickly outpaced Bennett's development. They easily sat up unassisted, took their first steps, clapped their hands, and jabbered their first words. We observed how easily the younger two were physically able to do things that Bennett would never be able to do. Those milestone moments continued to surprise us. The weight of the losses hit at unexpected times—most days we did not even realize how many losses we had lived through. But then the losses would hit us as we watched Jackson lie on the floor quietly on his back, roll over on his stomach, pop up onto all fours, and crawl across the room. A toddler's natural physical development was something we had not experienced due to Bennett's quadriplegic cerebral palsy diagnosis.

Pushing through the losses, it is a joy to watch our children grow and mature. As we had never heard Bennett say "mama" or "dada," Jackson and Reagan quickly started figuring out words like "NO!"

"MINE," and "I DO IT!" One day around the age of two, Reagan blurted, "Stop it, Mommy! You hurting my feelings!" My dad was sitting there in our armchair for a visit, and he almost fell out of his chair laughing when he heard her express her strong and insightful feelings. We went from a relatively quiet and calm house to a loud and opinionated house rapidly. One bustling fall evening I was in the kitchen attempting to get dinner on the table because the troops were hangry (*han*gry: bad-tempered or irritable as a result of hunger*). Reagan and Jackson were preschoolers, fighting over a toy, and their argument was ramping up. I stepped in to de-escalate their scuffle when Jackson screamed, "I want Bennett to talk!" We all froze at his surprising words. Silence filled the room, and all I could think was, "Out of the mouths of babes." God only knows why Jackson said that. Maybe he was sad that he was unable to talk with his brother? Maybe he was hoping Bennett would take "his side" in his duel with his little sister? Maybe he wished that Bennett could get disciplined for his actions, as Jackson was about to be. Regardless of his intention, Jackson put words to the deep loss we all felt that Bennett could not speak to us.

An event that encapsulates the craziness of our life was the day of the missed school bus drop-off. When Bennett was in second grade, his school bus would drop him off at our home around three-thirty in the afternoon. On a "great" day, the two younger kids would be both taking an afternoon nap together and on a "good" day at least one of them would be asleep at that time. One particularly *not so great day*, neither child (ages four and two), wanted to take a nap. I had finally gotten Reagan to fall asleep in her crib, and after a round of debate with Jackson, I agreed to lie on his floor next to his bed to help him to fall asleep. My head hit the carpet, and the next thing I knew I was waking up in a jolt of pure panic.

I had fallen into a deep sleep (preschool moms know the level of exhaustion I am talking about), it was an hour past Bennett's bus's drop-off time, and I was in complete freak-out mode. I darted down the stairs, looked out our front window to see if the bus was there waiting for me, but there was no bus. I then heard loud pounding on our back door, so I ran to the back of our house to find our beloved white-haired, elderly neighbor looking at me like I was crazy. "Where the hell have you been?" he asked me. "The bus has been here two times and I was about to knock this door down myself to find you. Are you okay?"

Bill is a retired Marine and a teddy bear with a heart of gold. I told him I was fine, grabbed my phone and started calling Bennett's school to see how I could find him. Much to my delight, the principal assured me Bennett was safe in her office—the bus had brought him back to school after coming to our house two times and not seeing an adult available to hand him off to. I then sped out the back door to our car, where Bill's feisty wife Coralie met me at the car asking, "Are you alright? What's wrong with you—have you been day drinking?" "NO!" I assured her, "I fell asleep trying to get the kids to take naps! Can you please stay with them for a few minutes while I run up to get Bennett from his school?" I am not sure that she believed me, but all I knew was that I had to go get my baby in the principal's office. She agreed and I was off.

I burst into the principal's office and found her smiling at me with Bennett next to her desk like an angel waiting in a wheelchair. I was embarrassed and tried to explain that my younger two kids would not nap, so I laid down with one, and the next thing I knew I had overslept the arrival of his bus. She kept smiling, nodded, and assured me that "things like this happen all the time." I was mortified and could not believe that this was happening. I was overcome with shame. I had always been so vigilant when it came to Bennett's needs and schedule, but this time I frankly blew it. I quickly thanked her over and over again, wheeled him out, kissed his soft cheeks and promised Bennett that would be his first and last visit to the principal's office.

When dreams don't come true

When Reagan was three years old, I was thrilled that she was finally old enough to sign up for a local community beginners' ballet class. Reagan had always walked around on her tippy toes (not a good thing, per numerous physical therapists' observations), and I had beamed and nodded at the many people who told us she looked like a little ballerina. I bought her a little pink leotard, matching pink skirt and tights, and soft ballet slippers for the big first day of class. When the crisp fall morning finally arrived, she excitedly got dressed, slipped on her ballet slippers, and was all set for our first class. I pulled her blond Shirley-Temple-like curls back into a tight bun, and we walked into the large open dance studio filled with little ones and their mothers or nannies.

The gorgeous ballet teacher had Swiss-chocolate-colored skin and a French accent as smooth as the finest wine. She called all her little ballerinas to the dance floor like a mother swan calling together all her little cygnets into a huddle. Reagan shook her head left to right and started backing into my legs. I was surprised, but I figured that after a few moments of watching all the other children line up and participate in the fun, she would surely join into the whirling, twirling, and leaping. I could not have been more wrong.

For the entire forty-five-minute class Reagan absolutely refused to join the class. As the instructor led the class in stretches and taught them first position, she pleasantly called out, "Reagan, come join your friends!" Reagan stood there stubbornly, pressed back hard into my legs, and forcefully stood her ground. She was not going to let a toe touch that wooden dance floor. We left the first class abruptly. I tried to ask questions about why she did not want to participate, but I could never get a real answer from the newly three-year-old. Surprise, surprise. All she knew was that she did not want to do it. For the next three weeks this continued. One day she actually decided to join the circle of children for stretching and did one leap across the floor, but quickly leapt right back to the waiting area where I sat. That was it; she refused to participate any more.

As a mother, I felt completely defeated and was very frustrated. I know it sounds silly, but I was confused as to why my one and only little girl, who had dressed up in tutus and twirled around the house gleefully, now hated ballet class. My expectations had been thrown out the window, money had been flushed down the toilet, and I was left staring at myself in the mirror, forced to ask myself why I was having such a hard time letting go of the introduction-to-ballet disaster.

I had not grown up taking dance classes. I started dancing in middle school, a decade later than most little girls I knew who had danced. My mom was the furthest thing from a "dance mom." She had never forced me to put on any form of costume or leotard, and I had never felt any pressure to perform to any certain standard. I did not feel I was "parenting out of my own woundedness," and yet I struggled to understand why my daughter refused to participate.

The bottom line was that she hated ballet class, and by week five I accepted the fact that I could not control or make this little person do something that she did not want to do. It was a profound moment in my motherhood journey because none of my pep talks or "positive parenting" techniques were working; plus my assumption that "All little girls love ballet" was smashed. I swiftly realized that lessons like this would only continue to be more and more prevalent as the years went on. My children are their own unique beings, filled with distinctive passions, talents, and interests. What was whispered into my heart then, and what has been confirmed through the years, was that my dreams for my kids may not be what comes true. And that is more than okay. The more I take the time to chase what it is that lights their hearts on fire, the more beautiful life is for all of us.

That being said, our middle son voiced to me one lazy summer day, "I don't feel like I matter." Such a middle-child thing to say, right? I have always loved studying birth-order theories, but no collegiate study gave me the answer to Jackson's raw reflection at the age of eight. That simple statement gutted me to my core because it flagged for us as parents that the ways we were seeking to connect with him at that time were not effective. I am so grateful that he had the words to attach to his feelings on that difficult summer day. He was opening his heart up to us and this was an opportunity for me as a mother to acknowledge that we needed to make some adjustments in our interactions with him. Being the sibling of a special-needs child is unique and presents unique feelings, circumstances, challenges, and losses. Parenting our three uniquely different children continues to keep us humble, re-evaluating what our "dreams" are, and clinging to hope that it will all work out.

He's fine! He's fine!

Our three children, born in a span of five years, each grew at different rates. Bennett was very small on his growth curve, Jackson was above average in his growth curve, and Reagan was off the charts on her growth curve. As a result, family outings in the early years required Bennett in his wheelchair, and the younger two strapped in a double stroller to keep them contained. Released from their five-point harnesses, they usually headed in opposite directions, so safety was always our number-one priority. Speaking of safety, Bennett's doctor had suggested that we get a handicap parking tag for our car to ensure that getting Bennett in and out of the car with his wheelchair provided the utmost safety for him. We reluctantly agreed, knowing that he would continue to grow to the point at which we would eventually need a handicap-accessible van.

After grueling days of child rearing, while changing the diapers of three children around the clock, every now and then we attempted to get out of the house with our six-, three-, and one-year-olds. If the weather was good, we would load up our family car for an outing of an early dinner and a walk to the park. Mexican food and margaritas were usually our palates' cravings. On a particularly warm yet pleasant summer night, we slowly pulled our family car into the parking garage and found a handicap parking space. After parking, Travis put the blue handicap parking tab on the car's rearview mirror, and we began the challenging task of unbuckling the three kids out of their car seats. It took the hand skills of Houdini to quickly unbuckle the younger two and immediately buckle them into the stroller's five-point harness (to keep them from wrestling free and darting across the parking garage). Sweaty armpits and chaotic maneuvering were the norm for those toddler-filled outings.

After unloading Bennett from the car and reloading him into his wheelchair alongside his three-year-old and one-year-old siblings strapped into their double jogger stroller, we each pushed one and started walking. We saw a woman in a wheelchair and a friend of hers coming toward the handicap spots. We had turned to walk to the restaurant when we heard yelling: "Hey! Hey! Hey you!" We looked around, assuming that we had dropped a pacifier, beloved blanket, or stuffed animal. Instead, we came face to face with a female senior citizen in the wheelchair screaming at us while shaking her finger. "You're not supposed to park there! This is illegal!" We defended ourselves by saying, "Oh, ma'am, we have a son with cerebral palsy and his doctor gave us the handicap tag to ensure his safety in parking lots." The woman in the wheelchair continued to scream while wheeling herself toward us, "He's fine! He's fine! He's just fine! Cerebral palsy has nothing on spina bifida!"

Her ranting continued with anger and vitriol, and her female friend stood there with a smile plastered on her face. At this point I honestly looked around thinking, "We must be on 'candid camera' right now. There must be a camera filming what our response will be to this angry woman. This has to be a setup." Our kids looked puzzled as she continued screaming at us like the Wicked Witch of the West in a wheelchair. Unfortunately, there were no cameras and this did not appear to be a joke. Trying to assess the situation I immediately saw Travis's red face and could almost see his blood pressure rising. Nothing we said calmed her, so we walked away and continued pushing our kids in their strollers toward the restaurant. I focused on the red brick wall leading us out of the parking garage. Instead of the Wizard of Oz's "Follow the Yellow Brick Road" tune going through our heads, it was more like "Follow the Red Brick Wall" to flee this appalling onslaught.

With each step taken away from the angry senior citizen, we were trembling with irritation. We wondered, "Is she going to slash our tires or key our car? We were parked there legally, so even if she called the police, would they come track us down?" Within ten minutes we were seated in the restaurant shaken, barely able to swallow our beloved chips and salsa. Our appetite had been ruined and yet our skin was thickened in that moment. Prior to that day, if a stranger approached us, we had grown accustomed to kind or encouraging words or reflections when they saw Bennett. This backward hostile experience showed us loud and clear that positive interactions regarding Bennett will not always be the norm. We also realized that discrimination is alive and well within the disability community.

The day of the parking-lot incident was an example of the pain in the human condition. Upon further reflection, it turned out to be a good teaching moment for us as parents. Years later we still use that example when talking to our kids about the simple truth that "hurt people hurt people." I will never forget the bitterness and rage that spewed from that dear old soul in the parking garage. After that experience I pledged to myself to never allow my pain to fester into a toxic rage toward another human being. The woman's physical disabilities were no doubt extremely painful, limiting, and agonizing. I would never pretend to understand what it is like to live a day in her body. And yet at the same time, it felt as if she did not care to see Bennett for who he is. How could she know what he suffered from on a daily basis, with no ability to speak, share, or verbalize his pain? She certainly did not take the time to recognize the challenges that we experienced in our daily care of him as well as his two younger siblings. Deep gut-wrenching pain is a universal condition. It is the one thing that we are all guaranteed to experience at some point in our lives. It has been our experience, as we cross paths with all types of hurting people, that the more grace (not judgement) we extend to those we come across, the more peace we have in our own lives.

Sometimes that is easier said than done. Back when Bennett was a toddler, numerous well-meaning, kind folks said to us, "Oh, how sweet! He's sleeping." We wanted to respond with, "Actually he is wide awake but does not have the strength to hold his head up." Similarly, one day an old man walked up to me when Bennett was old enough to appear "non-typical," and in an effort to prepare me for the future, he got close to my face, looked me in the eyes, and informed me, "You have no idea how many people are going to make fun of him as he grows up because he looks so funny. But God will take care of them once they die!" Wow. Bizarre encounters have become par for our course.

CHAPTER 17

Respite, Jill's House, and Childcare

Respite: a short period of rest or relief from something difficult or unpleasant.

BENNETT HAD RECENTLY turned three years old when we left Tennessee and moved back to the Washington, D.C., area. We were a young couple in our thirties with two young boys, one with special needs and the other due to be born any day. We knew we wanted a strong faith community for our boys to be spiritually formed. Travis and I each grew up in churches that felt filled with extended family members, and we longed for our boys to have that same experience.

The first Sunday that we visited a large, well-known church in Northern Virginia, we sat in the service with Bennett in his stroller next to us and Jackson still "cooking" in my stomach. It was a much larger church than we had ever attended, the music and sermon were incredible, and the experience of the church felt like stepping into a well-oiled machine. It had a ministry for every need imaginable, including a ministry for kids with special needs, called "Access." We wanted to learn more about Access, because we had never left Bennett in a nursery so that we might attend a worship service as a couple. Bennett had always come with us. On that very day though, at the end of the service, the pastor stood on the stage with several others to announce and dedicate the opening of "Jill's House." We had not heard of Jill's House before, but our attention was quickly sparked as they went on to describe that numerous private donors had donated more than $13 million to build a facility to provide overnight respite to children with disabilities.

Studies have shown that more than 80 percent of marriages with a special-needs child end in divorce, not to mention a list of stresses including depression, anxiety, financial crisis, and hopelessness. The Jill's House founders, Lon and Brenda Solomon, knew the pain of caring for a daughter, Jill, with severe disabilities, and after traveling to a respite home in Israel they came back to the United States and decided to raise funds to build a comparable facility here. Jill's House is the first overnight respite care facility of its kind in America. After word got out about the mission of Jill's House, support and donors came flooding in as people recognized this unique opportunity to support these children and families in a powerful and transformative way.

As we watched the group on the stage humbly announce, dedicate, and pray over Jill's House, Travis and I knew in our hearts that we had found the faith community for us. They looked at our family, most especially our precious son Bennett, and boldly declared that his life matters. We also felt this was a safe place for us to strengthen our faith while finding support, encouragement, and strength for our journey as Bennett's parents and caregivers. We left church that day feeling overcome with gratitude and hope for the exciting possibilities that lay ahead if we committed to attending this very special church.

In the weeks following that first Sunday visit, we enrolled Bennett in Sunday school through the Access ministry. When we dropped him off each Sunday, he was greeted by a trained teacher as well as a staff nurse (!) to care for him for the hour and a half that we participated in the worship service. The initial Sunday in October, sitting in the church's large auditorium without Bennett (I was still pregnant with Jackson) felt extremely odd. It was a feeling we will never forget. We knew he was in loving, safe care, so we attempted to take a deep breath, relax, and soak in the worship experience.

In the years to follow, we regularly attended weekly services, our three kids attended Sunday school with nurturing and loving teachers, and we were extremely blessed by the community. We were particularly blessed to get to know the small group of Access volunteers who consistently cared for Bennett each week. These dedicated volunteers knew which toys would make him giggle and which toys would make him scream. They surrounded our family with acceptance, love, and support week in and week out.

Let me be clear. We were a loud and dramatic traveling circus back in those days as we were juggling toddlers, calming tantrums, and changing endless diapers. But as we look back, they were joyous, messy, and treasured times. The love shown to our family through the Access ministry we will never forget. Because our first child had come into the world in a completely non-typical fashion, we were thrown into years feeling anything but normal. We were used to looks of sympathy or unease, but finally through Access, and later Jill's House, we had found community with people who "got" us, valued us, and were not too offended by the "Hot Mess Express" that we were.

Soon after Bennett turned seven, he spent his first weekend at Jill's House. He had never spent a night away from both Travis and me. We had each established a night away from Bennett to meet with a group of college girl or guy friends, but in seven years Travis and I had not had one weekend "away together." Jill's House requires that parents select a weekend preference on a quarterly basis, so the weekend we signed up for included Travis's thirty-seventh birthday. We had plans to settle the younger two kids with my mom on that Saturday, head to a hotel, dine out, sleep, swim, and try to relax—something that was quite frankly foreign to us. We did not know how to begin the process of unwinding the tightly-wound ball of yarn that was our past stressful seven years.

As I packed up Bennett's bag, gathering all his clothes, diapers, wipes, medical supplies, formula, prescriptions, and favorite toys, feelings of guilt, dread, and panic came over me. What were we doing? What were we thinking? How could we leave him for two nights with complete strangers? What if he had a seizure? What if he choked on his formula and they didn't see him choking? In my head I knew we were not being selfish for taking Bennett to Jill's House. They had a full-time nurse caring for him, trained fellows, and a doctor on call at all times. And yet my heart wrestled with the fact that caring for Bennett was *my* job and I was having a hard time handing him over. I knew every move he made, every sound that came out of his body. I could tell the minute a sickness was settling in his lungs by the gurgle of his breathing or number of coughs.

And yet this was the time and the safe place to let Bennett take baby steps into the care of others. He had been attending school for four years, had been under the care of other professionals for years, and was doing great. Any guilt or grief that I had was completely normal, and yet my marriage with Travis needed to be a priority. This was the perfect time to seize this opportunity and go celebrate my man's thirty-seventh birthday. We rolled Bennett into Jill's House on that dark autumn night, we stopped in front of the large roaring fireplace (Jill's House is designed to look like a cozy ski lodge), and we gave him kisses goodbye. Bennett looked around, probably wondering what in the world was going on, but his sweet attendant quickly vocalized for him, "Bye, Mom! Bye, Dad! Have a great first respite weekend!" And off he went.

My heartstrings tugged as we walked through the sliding doors to exit Jill's House. Travis and I quickly hopped into our car, and when I sat down my stomach hurt and a few tears slipped down my cheeks. It was hard to leave Bennett, but the weekend away with Travis was spectacular and much needed. When we picked Bennett up from Jill's House on Sunday afternoon, he was calm, smiling, and peaceful. He had swum, played, and been doted on all weekend long. They gave us a written summary of all the activities and interactions he had experienced during his forty-eight hours at Jill's House. The gift of respite was like honey to his soul (and ours) and continues to be to this day.

Through the years we have become involved with fundraising for Jill's House, and through word of mouth and generous giving there are now Jill's House respite locations across the United States. We always say that if you are looking for a cause to support that literally changes lives for good—guaranteed—then look no further (www.jillshouse. org). Their level of care for children with disabilities and their families has become a new standard of excellence that many now come to visit, study, and then return to their cities to replicate. Our younger two children have even become involved in their "siblings night" quarterly gatherings, and it has become a highlight for them, too, to now "get to go to Jill's House."

One definition of the word "respite" means "to relieve temporarily, especially from anything distressing or trying; give an interval of relief from." Parents of children with disabilities are not special. They are simply parents who love their children. Sometimes loving and caring for their children is exponentially more difficult than caring for a "normal" child, demanding more patience, more self-control, more research, more medical interventions, and more support. This is where Jill's House has come in and said to families, "Your child has dignity and worth, and we want to care for them to the fullest of our abilities.

We want you parents to rest, sleep, go for a walk, go out to eat, spend time with your other kids, or just enjoy some alone time."

Respite has been a gift that we did not realize we needed until our house was quiet, empty, and still, and there was no responsibility except to tap into our hearts and see what self-care was needed. Sometimes we have spent a weekend alone, other times we have planned social gatherings, and other times we have done a quick weekend trip for recreational companionship. Regardless of what we spend the weekend doing, we know that Bennett is swimming, on the playground, being sung to, and playing with friends with nonstop attention being poured over him.

Jill's House restored hope in our hearts that we had people on this earth who valued and adored Bennett almost as much as we do. The Jill's House weekend respite experiences have confirmed that we are not alone on this day-in-and-day-out journey that at times feels somewhat monotonous—eerily close to the mornings in the 1993 film *Groundhog Day* with Bill Murray. One nurse in particular, Courtney, always sent notes home with Bennett telling us how special he is, offering to help us out if we were ever in need of additional care at home. Courtney's small, unexpected notes were a great gift and confirmed to us that Bennett's life does matter, that he is not alive by chance or coincidence. Courtney saw something in Bennett that we and our family members and friends are continually drawn to: the purest form of innocence, truly a miracle you can see, touch, and hear.

Jill's House has blessed each member of our family with weekend respite, siblings' pizza parties, fabulous golf tournaments, incredible seats cheering on our Washington Nationals baseball team, festive Christmas parties, and even tickets to the White House Easter Egg Roll in the spring of 2017. It is a gift to be a part of the Jill's House family.

Our first hired babysitter

Through the years we have interviewed and hired babysitters for our children, because Travis works full-time and I have worked in both full-time and part-time positions. Gigi first entered our house to interview with us when Bennett was three and Jackson was two months old. I was attempting to return to the employer I had been working for full-time when Bennett was born, and they had graciously offered me an opportunity to come back on a part-time basis. We had never interviewed a nanny, so we Googled "what interview questions to ask during a nanny interview" and greeted her at the door with big smiles, healthy skepticism, and inviting postures.

Beginner's luck is truly a "thing" because we hit the jackpot with Gigi. I could immediately tell that Gigi was honest, trustworthy, an experienced mother of an eight-year-old daughter, and it was more than clear that she truly loved children. She had a sister back in Ethiopia with disabilities, and she talked about her sister with such love and affection that my gut told me she had to be our nanny.

All my instincts were confirmed when Jackson woke up from his nap, I handed him to Gigi, and she was completely taken with him and he with her. Gigi was immediately hired after I phoned her references and prayed that they all had strong recommendations, which they did. There began our strong bond with her and her family, an unlikely relationship that continues on to this day. We have shared birthdays, baby showers, struggles and joys with Gigi and her family, and we know she was an angel sent from above, because very few people would have felt comfortable with caring for our boys.

There are many beautiful things about Gigi. For one thing, she is stunningly beautiful. But more beautiful than the outer beauty is the beauty of her spirit, character, and heart deep within. She has always had the sweetest and most honest demeanor. If something was not right, she spoke up. If Jackson threw up every time he ate green beans, she would tell me to stop feeding him the green beans I left out for her to feed him. We have laughed a lot with her during the years she spent watching our boys. We never worried when the boys were in her care. We fully admit that she basically taught us how to have a nanny as we welcomed her into our "crazy." We gratefully appreciated Gigi's willingness to join our wild ride and have continued our relationship with her for more than ten years.

Gigi and her family are a beautiful example of hardworking, principled, family-oriented people chasing the American Dream. Gigi and her husband have two beautiful, smart, and talented daughters who are absolutely delightful. The sky is the limit for these two girls, and I deeply respect the fact that their parents have worked vigorously to provide them every opportunity available. From story time at local libraries to swimming lessons and new sports experiences, their girls are given every possible opportunity to chase their dreams. Their faith is also extremely important to them. Gigi lost her father when she was very young, traveled from Ethiopia to Dubai seeking work, and met her now-husband there. Gigi's husband was raised very humbly by his mother in Ethiopia, who helped to keep house for US diplomats serving there.

One of the best days of my adult life was when Gigi was pregnant with her second daughter, and I had asked for a list of her friends to throw her an "American baby shower." She had given me a guest list. My mom and I gathered all the food and decorations and we set everything up in Gigi's dining room for easy access for her neighbors and nearby friends. The room was bustling with excitement and love for the new arrival soon joining Gigi's family.

As I was greeting the guests and taking gifts to the back room, I was stopped and hugged by an older woman whom I did not know. She whispered to me, "I am Jenny, and I knew Gigi's husband when he was a young boy." This woman was a US diplomat's wife. Jenny was overjoyed to attend the baby shower for the "little boy" she used to know. I was blown away by the "small world" we live in, and my heart was full that day as Gigi's house filled with female chatter and laughter. Women from all across the world sat in chairs and couches lining the walls. We shared food, watched her open her gifts, and each told stories of motherhood. There were Christians, Jews, and Muslims, whites and blacks, Nigerians and Ethiopians, mothers, aunts, sisters, daughters, and children, and Gigi was showered with love by all of them. Watching Gigi radiantly beam that day was a gift. The hope poured out through these lives, both old and new, and relationships joined together from around the world, are powerful—and indescribable. Gigi was our babysitter because she was comfortable caring for children with special needs; that qualification led her to us, but now she had become so much more than a babysitter.

CHAPTER 18
Hospitalizations and Surgeries

"If we have no peace, it's because we have forgotten
that we belong to each other."
— Mother Teresa

A S BENNETT'S BONES GREW, his stiffened muscles
pulled on his bones, and unfortunately the outcome is
quite negative. A common issue for kids with quadriplegic
cerebral palsy is that their hip "balls and sockets" get out
of whack. Bennett's muscles were daily pulling on his leg bones, tug-
ging so consistently that eventually his leg bones were slipping out of
his hip sockets. Add to this the fact that these kids are typically not
walking around consistently, giving the bones and muscles the impact
they were created to absorb, so eventually the topic of orthopedic surgery comes up. When Bennett was around seven years old his hips
were out of alignment, so we went for an orthopedic consultation. The
doctor very flippantly told us that routine surgery should go into both
hips, place plates in his bones, screw everything into place, and he
would be in a body cast for six weeks. Then he should be all set to go.

As a mother, the words "body cast for six weeks" was a horrific phrase to hear. I would have been horrified even for my typical children, but the thought of Bennett having a seizure or a choking spell while wearing a body cast was more than I could fathom. We took that information, and then sought a second opinion. It is no coincidence that during this time we had been weekly driving out to a local farm in the rolling hills of northern Virginia's wine country. Bennett was doing equine therapy at this farm, which consisted of placing him in the saddle on the back of a horse to increase his core strength. The lessons were a refuge for our entire family as we walked around the grounds, soaking up the beauty and peace that we found in the green lush grass, red barns, and magnificent historical houses.

The farm's owners have a truly remarkable family and a deeply inspiring story as to how they got started having therapeutic horseback riding for kids with disabilities. One spring day after Bennett had wrapped up his therapy lesson, in passing we mentioned our concern about his hips. Mark, the owner of the farm, stopped us as we were loading up our car and said, "Oh, you must visit Children's Hospital of Philadelphia (CHOP) in Pennsylvania. I will contact the surgeon we use there. He is the very best, and he does not require body casts. There are other less invasive procedures available for children like ours." We were beyond relieved to hear this news and had an appointment scheduled in Philadelphia within a week.

Bennett had a leg muscle lengthening surgery in the summer of 2014 at CHOP, and then three years later, in June 2017, a more involved double hip surgery at Johns Hopkins University Hospital in Baltimore. As he grew, his lower extremities were requiring medical interventions, and we did our best to take the advice of doctors at the top of their fields. The surgeries and recoveries were not easy, and the surgery in June 2017 at Johns Hopkins created the most challenging summer in our family's story to date. What started off as a double hip procedure to screw the hip bones into their sockets (a very non-medical way to put it) ended up as another ongoing nightmare.

We had the utmost confidence in our world-renowned surgeon, who immediately gave us his cellphone number and answered after the first ring whenever we called. His attention to X-ray details, his bedside manner, and his unwavering commitment to Bennett (and thousands of other children) leave us with nothing but the utmost respect for this man. His skilled hands performed the particularly lengthy surgery as he and his team restructured both of Bennett's hip sockets and bone alignments impeccably. He came out of the operating room one evening in May 2017 reporting to us that the surgery had gone well, Bennett had lost a lot of blood but did not require a blood transfusion, and that we could see him in the recovery room shortly.

As Bennett was recovering from the surgery in his bright, sun-filled room at Hopkins, a handsome young surgeon came to do rounds and check on him. We were told that everything looked fantastic, to keep the pain meds going for a few days after we were home, but that the recovery should be like clockwork—plus he shared the great news that we could go home the next day. I was apprehensive about transferring Bennett from wheelchair to bed, when to bathe him, and so on, so when I inquired about how careful we needed to be, the surgeon gave me a big George Clooney *ER* smile and replied, "Those hips are screwed in so tight, they are not coming out! Aside from accidentally dropping him to the ground, those screws are not going anywhere." I breathed a big sigh of relief, encouraged that we were up for the task of his rehabilitation at home.

Unfortunately, things did not go as smoothly at home as we were hoping. Around week two, Bennett started screaming in agonizing pain. He had run out of his pain meds and we had not refilled them because he "should not have needed them any longer." When the ongoing wails continued we were concerned, but assumed it was the healing process. When his left incision opened up and oozed, we notified the surgeon and they immediately said to come in for X-rays. The worst-case scenario had occurred: The plate from his left hip had slipped out from the bone, it was infected, and the surgeon had to open him back up to perform a revision surgery. Bennett was immediately placed on strong antibiotics to fight the raging infection which had caused the oozing.

Upon learning all this I simply burst into tears. The tears probably represented exhaustion and anger mixed with trauma from his birth ten years prior. I could not believe he was going back in for emergency surgery. I immediately called Travis, who was home with our younger two children, and he made childcare plans so he could be in Baltimore that night for the surgery. Travis arrived at the hospital around dinnertime, we fell into each others' arms, and made our way to the surgical waiting room. We sat typing on our laptops trying to make the time pass, anxiously waiting to hear how the revision surgery was going. Finally, and once again, our beloved surgeon came out and said that surgery had gone well. He was able to scrape out the infection inside the left incision site, and he emphasized that he was very sorry this revision surgery had been deemed necessary. Bennett had done remarkably well, was resting peacefully, and we could soon come to see him in recovery.

Because the surgery was unexpected and not scheduled, it had begun late, finishing up well after midnight. Travis and I had sat alone in the waiting area, the darkness of the night encompassing the large windows; the stillness of the usually bustling hospital sent chills down our spines. As we walked into the recovery area to see our precious son—once again, ten years later, our baby boy was lying on a white sheet, his skin almost as white as the sheets, his lips chapped from the dry air of the operating room. He had lost a lot of blood, but the surgeon told us that he had not required a blood transfusion. That was a relief, and yet we still were sad that once again our little fighter had experienced a less-than-ideal outcome from what should have been a somewhat routine double hip corrective surgery.

There is no way to sugarcoat what a setback this second surgery was to Travis and me individually and as a couple. We did not see it coming, the second surgery felt like an assault on our cores, and it left us completely going through the motions of life. Shower. Brush teeth. Take turns going home to sleep and be with the younger two kids. Thank the family members and friends sweeping in to feed us and care for us. I was not necessarily mad at God, but my feelings were hurt. Watching our son suffer repeatedly was scraping away at our hearts, shaking us in ways that were different. We were very short with each other. We had developed skepticism regarding what the medical professionals were telling us. The joy seemed unreachable. The future seemed much murkier. Yet we pushed through.

Bennett made positive strides in weaning off the strong pain meds, tolerating his formula tube feedings, and was deemed ready to go home. We were cautiously optimistic, so upon discharge part two, we assured the kind nurses that we were handling Bennett as delicately as possible, like a rose petal, and praying that we did not have to make another visit to Johns Hopkins Hospital for a very long time.

That wish would not come true, much to our disappointment. Bennett had spent most of the summer of 2017 lying down to heal those hips, and his bones had become very brittle due to lack of weight-bearing activities such as standing upright in a stander or gait trainer. Bone density is crucial for all of us, and the bones of kids like Bennett who do not stand and walk do not get the impact that a typical child's bones get. We had been eager to take him back to physical therapy to allow him to stand up in a standing device or gait trainer, but it was a slow process because we had to ensure his healing was complete before he could return to physical therapy.

Much to our dismay, before he could get back to school in the fall of 2017, Bennett's legs developed two small hairline fractures that were exceptionally painful. His screaming and sensitivity to touch told us that something was very wrong. It was grueling to watch him be in pain with no way to fully express what was hurting him. We do not know how the fractures happened. Perhaps merely rolling him over to change his diaper or clothes or transferring him to his wheelchair caused them. We shook with fear at the thought that our son's healing was so delicate that a mere caregiving gesture could be the instigator of devastating pain.

With the first fracture, before knowing what his intense pain was stemming from, I drove to the emergency room in tears, begging God to show His mercy on our son. If the metal plate had slid out from his hip again, requiring a third surgery, I was quite sure I was going to scream and melt into a puddle of defeat on the ER floor. We pulled up to the ER about nine o'clock in the evening, realizing that I had no wheelchair for Bennett with me (this was before we owned a wheel-chair-accessible van). I ran into the ER where there were a few families sitting in the chairs, and frantically said to the triage nurse, "I have my son in the car screaming in pain, but I don't have his wheelchair and I need a stretcher!" The nurse, startled, called for backup, and they came out with a wheelchair for me to transfer Bennett into and wheel him back for X-rays immediately.

Earlier that evening I had already spoken with our beloved sur-geon. In fact he was the one who asked me to bring Bennett in. He was deeply concerned and assured me that he would meet us there, no matter how late I arrived. Bennett was quickly registered in the ER and lay on the table screaming in pain while they took X-rays of his hips and legs from multiple angles. I watched his face wince with pain as he wept, and once again, I stood like a shell of complete helplessness. *Please, God. Please make this stop. How much more does this child have to endure?* We were placed in a room to wait for the X-ray results. Bennett was so exhausted from it all that he lay on the bed limp, his eyes watching his favorite *Wiggles* show on my phone as we attempted to pass the time. Time in a hospital almost always feels like a time warp or the twilight zone where minutes, hours, and days seem to ooze together like a dense pile of sticky slime.

The surgeon walked into the room where we waited and was initially baffled. The X-rays showed that Bennett's hips were healing beautifully, just as he expected them to look at this point in the healing process. He examined Bennett's legs gently, attempting to ascertain the exact place where the pain was coming from, but Bennett would not allow him to touch or move anything without deafening wailing. As a result, orders were placed for new X-rays focusing on the lower extremities, and finally around midnight he had figured out there was a slight hairline fracture on Bennett's left leg, his weaker side, just above the knee in his femur. This fracture did not require surgery or a cast, only a leg brace to keep his left leg straight and still. There was not much more that we could do other than to keep his leg stationary, give him over-the-counter pain meds, and ensure that Bennett was getting enough calcium. Another small fracture happened again later in the fall of 2017, but thankfully with each small fracture the healing occurred swiftly and the leg brace became his new accessory as he went to school.

The summer of 2017 stretched us in ways that we did not know we had room to be stretched. The stress levels of caring for Bennett, along with his seven- and five-year-old siblings, took a lot of energy, not to mention the strain on our marriage. The continuous medical complications required constant logistical communication, yet we barely ever had any real time to process any of our feelings together. Weeks of stress led to stuffed feelings, rising tensions, bad coping mechanisms, and eventually a very frank conversation. It was determined that we needed to see a marriage counselor immediately. I felt abandoned at times; Travis felt overwhelmed with the chore of providing for all our needs. It was time to call in a professional's help.

We searched for a therapist near us, finding a very experienced one not too far from where we lived, and scheduled an appointment as soon as she was available. She was exactly what we needed at that time, and we highly recommend seeking out the help of marriage counselors when you face stressful times. Sitting in that counselor's office we were able to find peace, calm, and validation for the stress that we were managing. I will never forget when the counselor looked at us after hearing all that we had been juggling for the past ten years and said to us, "Do you realize that your marriage is under assault?" No one had ever stated it like that, but she put words to exactly what we had been feeling. Words of validation are a truly remarkable thing to one's psyche. We were able to work through some frustrations that each of us had been bottling up and found a way to navigate through that very difficult chapter in our story, the summer of 2017.

Night nurses

Parents of children with disabilities know that accessing state-funded medical assistance programs is grueling. There were waitlists for everything. In fact, we applied for the Maryland Medicaid waiver when Bennett was three years old, and he did not get "approved" until the age of ten—seven years later. We spent years waiting to move up one to three spots per year, depending on how many kids listed ahead of us had passed away (morbid, but true). The endless paperwork was frustrating, the process was maddening, and we were exhausted, all at the same time.

Finally, in the fall of 2017, after Bennett's double hip surgeries at Hopkins and the numerous complications that came from that, we were approved for the Maryland Model Waiver. Bennett's overnight formula feeds administered through his feeding tube plus the wound care required for his incisions had finally gained us approval for financial assistance. For years we had lived paycheck to paycheck as we paid the large out-of-pocket costs for Bennett's hypoallergenic formula, doctor co-pays, surgical procedures, a wheelchair, a stander, a gait trainer, and a supported seating system. Our medical insurance usually covered a percentage, yet sometimes did not, so we spent a lot of time appealing for their help, but regardless, we always received substantial bills for which we were responsible.

It was shocking and yet a real relief when we realized we would finally have state assistance to help pay for the large expenses required to care for Bennett. Our personal health insurance was the first provider, and then anything not covered was paid for by Maryland Medicaid. Included in this program was overnight nursing in our house each night, from 11 p.m. to 7 a.m., to oversee Bennett's overnight tube feedings, care for him, and ensure that we, his caregivers, were given eight hours of solid sleep.

Prior to the Model Waiver authorization, we had functioned for ten years with no professional home nursing. We had experienced the amazing African nun, Nurse Ann, right after NICU discharge for an hour per week, but after we moved to Virginia, Tennessee, and back to Maryland, we had been on our own. We had basically been winging it. We had taught ourselves how to unclog formula feeding bags, how to re-insert feeding tube buttons (when they fell out, leaving a hole into his stomach), and how to keep all his syringes and breathing treatment equipment clean and reusable. Our sleep deprivation was real, and the thought of eight hours of rest while a nurse cared for Bennett was inconceivable. Yet the next challenge would be finding a few night nurses we would be comfortable with having in our house overnight.

We had interviewed babysitters before, but interviewing overnight nurses turned out to be an even bigger task. We needed to find individuals who were skilled, compassionate, and people we would be comfortable having in our house overnight while we were asleep. We were so very grateful for the opportunity and yet it all felt very uncomfortable at the same time. Whom did we want to see us in our pajamas, watch us get a midnight snack from the refrigerator, and trust to care for our son's every need, especially on the nights he was awake with fever, vomiting, or experiencing respiratory distress, normal occurrences that we had handled for the past ten years?

The first three candidates were sweet women, and although I am sure they are wonderful, they did not feel like the right fit. One ended up hanging out at our house for hours because her son could not come and get her, so I fed her a sandwich and we small-talked all about her life. Another worked a few shifts for us but seemed overly obsessed with my other two children, their toys and belongings, and frankly gave me a weird feeling. She worked a few shifts but made me feel as if I were entering into a relationship similar to that in the movie *The Hand That Rocks the Cradle*. Another nurse put Bennett to sleep, and then stood outside my house on her phone screaming at family members, so much that it woke my next-door neighbors up. After these first three nurses assigned to us, we were not too sure this "overnight nursing" situation would provide any respite. It felt more like another part-time job of managing personalities and expectations. In our house. Overnight. While we were supposed to be "resting."

But then the heavens opened, the clouds parted, and down floated a special nurse sent to us from above. The nursing manager told us, "I do have this one special nurse named Moji. She does not have a lot of availability, but I feel she could be a good fit for your family." Moji walked into our house, gave us her big, warm smile while she stood and stroked Bennett's hand, and my heart told me that we had found the right nurse. Through some schedule shifting, we were blessed to secure Moji as our Monday-Friday overnight nurse, and our lives have been incredibly enriched.

Moji is a very wise woman. She has seen much. She has lived far away from family, separated by oceans. Growing up in Nigeria, she attended church and sang songs such as "Nothing But the Blood of Jesus" and "Victory in Jesus"—two hymns that Travis and I grew up singing as well. One night I heard her humming the tune to "What can wash away my sins? Nothing but the blood of Jesus" while she was washing out Bennett's syringes. I stopped her and said, "Moji, I know that song!" We then joined in together singing familiar hymns, laughing, clapping, swaying, and sharing the common bond that only the body of Christ can cultivate across national borders.

Two women from very different backgrounds, countries, races, and traditions immediately held tight to a bond that no one could ever take from us. Our shared faith sealed our friendship, and I can honestly say that she is a dear and treasured friend. We text each other all the time; she sends me beautiful text memes for Mothers' Day, Christmas, Easter, and most holidays in between. When I am worried about Bennett, she is the first person I contact to hear her voice of calm. She is always saying at night while she stands at our sink, "Glory be to God in the highest! He is seated on His throne. We thank You, Father, for being so good to us. All will be well." Amen.

Seizures

In addition to Bennett's hips, bones, and lungs, Bennett's seizures are a beast of their own. The brain is one of the most complex organs in our bodies. Bennett's seizures began before he was one year old, and we did not get them fully medicated until he was almost three, when the neurologist in Nashville finally found the medication combination that worked for his brain damage. Since then we have had to increase his medicine dosages as he grew, but his seizures are for the most part controlled quite well.

There have been two large seizures during which he went limp, was unable to track with his eyes, and his right hand pulsated rhythmically, like a glitching TV screen. In each of these circumstances we were forced to call 911. In September of 2018, one of these "incidents" occurred while our family had been out for a walk together. The swampy summer air had been replaced with our first crisp, dry burst of fall air, and I recall walking through our neighborhood with my husband and three kids content and grateful for all I had been given. A few moments later I looked down at Bennett and saw that his eyes were "stuck" and not tracking. I told Travis, literally ran while pushing his chair home, administered extra doses of meds, and could quickly tell that we needed an ambulance. He was breathing but the breathing was shallow.

As I ran out the back door carrying Bennett limp in my arms, I passed Travis and our two younger children coming up the driveway. Their eyes were big, their little voices asking if he was okay, and we assured them that he was going to be okay, but we needed to get him to the hospital for a doctor to give him some medicine. They trustfully took our word for it and headed into the house. This was their "normal," and they did not know any differently. They have an older brother who visits doctors a lot, sits in a wheelchair, and cannot speak, walk, or eat by mouth. He has surgeries and braces and hospitalizations, and it all is just part of their "normal" life. It has caused us sadness to think that such small humans were faced with such hard realities, and yet we are extremely proud of the ways they always adapt and show the resiliency that children are known for.

At Children's National Hospital that evening the emergency room doctor doused Bennett with seizure meds, his seizure finally lifted, and Bennett and I both passed out asleep in our ER room (as we waited for a room to open up in the hospital). Much to my surprise, around 4 a.m. I was awakened by a tall, male medical fellow saying into my face, "Ms. Speck, Ms. Speck, you may go home now. We are discharging Bennett as he appears to be fine and there are no open beds in the hospital. Please call us if you have any issues once you are settled at home." I was stunned because 1) it was 4 a.m.; 2) I had no car (the ambulance had brought us); 3) Travis would have to wake up our two little kids, if I was even able to get him to answer his phone); and 4) my parents were each living in Virginia and the thought of waking either of them up at 4 a.m. to drive into D.C. to then take us home to Maryland seemed much too much to ask.

As I quickly tried to wake up and troubleshoot this ER nightmare, I told the kind fellow that we had no car and no one available to pick us up. I knew that was not his problem, but I was having a difficult time understanding how they could throw us into the street before the sun was even up. I had told Travis around midnight that we were being admitted to the hospital for observation, so he went to bed thinking we were safe and sound with a plan. "Well, you can call an Uber, ma'am. We have patients do that all the time," the fellow replied. *Wow. What is happening right now? Bennett cannot sit up on his own. I will have to hold him in the back seat. How am I going to find an Uber at four a.m. in Northeast D.C.? Is this even safe?*

By this point it felt as if I had no other choice, so I clicked on my Uber app, found a driver with a van that could fit us both, and the app told me he would be there in fifteen minutes. I asked to be discharged quickly, the paperwork was processed, they wheeled Bennett and me out to the ER entrance (with Bennett on my lap in the wheelchair), and by 5 a.m., before sunrise, we were driving along the pothole-filled streets of D.C. with a kind yet quiet Uber driver who shared that he was a husband and father of three children. I held on tightly to Bennett over every bump, watching each street sign as we wove through the dark alleys, and prayed the entire way as we headed toward our house.

After we walked in the door and turned on the light, Travis leapt up out of our bed thinking I was a ghost or a thief. He was completely shocked to see us. We hugged, I gave him a brief explanation of our abrupt discharge plus 5 a.m. Uber ride, and we both just shook our heads. It was further confirmation that our life is an ongoing saga, this episode landing us at the mercy of a compassionate immigrant who as the provider for a wife and three children was willing to pick up a mother and her disabled son from the emergency room. The driver had calmly talked to me, watched through his rearview mirror as Bennett lay over my lap in the back seat of his minivan, saw that Bennett could not sit up independently or speak, pulled up to the bottom of our driveway, and patiently watched as I delicately exited his minivan.

The sun was just beginning to rise over the trees that morning as I carried Bennett up our steep asphalt driveway. While the entire night in the ER felt like a bizarre dream, not once did I feel alone or abandoned. Rather, I had been sustained by the hope that the Creator of the sun I was watching rise from the east had us in His hands the entire time. And thinking of all that could have happened to us along the alleys of Northeast Washington D.C. in the dark of the night, He most certainly held on to us tightly, delivering us safely home via a vessel driven by a kind Uber driver.

CHAPTER 19
COVID-19

"Fear not, for I am with you."
— Isaiah 41:10
Bennett's hospitalization – March 2020

I N EARLY MARCH of 2020, I took a weekend trip to Charleston, South Carolina, planned with two dear college friends. We barely see each other thanks to the craziness of life, three husbands, and nine children, but every three to five years we make the effort. This was a trip I was extremely excited about. COVID-19 had grabbed the headlines of every news report during the week leading up to the trip. It was the week that the United States was shutting down events such as March Madness and international travel to and from China, then Europe. I wrestled internally with whether or not to even go, but Travis insisted that I make the trip.

Following the best available guidance at the time, I hopped on the plane to Charleston, South Carolina, and spent a weekend talking late into the night, eating delicious Southern cuisine, and walking up and down the gorgeous beaches discussing all things midlife with my friends.

My plane landed back home on Sunday evening, March 15, 2020, at Baltimore-Washington Airport. I was incredibly excited to see my family, anxiously awaiting the sight of our silver handicap-accessible van. When Travis and the kids pulled up, I gave Travis, Jackson, and Reagan hugs and kisses, and then hopped into the back of the van to kiss Bennett. As I leaned over to kiss his soft cheek, I immediately could tell that he was having trouble breathing. When I had left on that previous Friday, he had had a drippy nose from what I thought were his horrible seasonal allergies. But I immediately realized he had a full-blown virus that Travis had been managing (and not mentioning to me so that I would have fun and not worry). My mama bear instinct knew it was not good, but I tried hard to not let myself panic. Yet.

We got home, started doing around-the-clock breathing treatments and hot steamy showers, and Bennett actually slept well that first night back at home. When we woke up the next morning, Bennett was fighting the virus, and at midday none of our respiratory "tricks" were working to calm his breathing. By March 16, 2020, our kids' schools and Travis's workplace had all "shut down," so we were all at home together. Bennett was in respiratory distress but I did not want to panic and set off alarm bells in the house, so I gingerly walked down our beige-carpeted basement stairs to Travis's home "office" to tell him we had to take Bennett to the hospital. He was quickly getting worse, not better. Travis ran upstairs to see him, agreed, and after a quick heated discussion regarding who would take him, we decided that I would. Travis would stay home with the two younger kids so that they could have a "normal" evening and bedtime. We have an oximeter that monitors Bennett's oxygen levels, and his levels were decent, hanging out in the mid- 90s, so I did not feel we needed an ambulance. Instead I loaded Bennett into our van and we quickly headed for Children's National Hospital in Washington, D.C.

As I drove Bennett along the pothole-ridden streets of D.C., it hit me that he could have COVID-19. I called his night nurse Moji to let her know, and she told me that everything was going to be okay and that I was doing the right thing. Simply hearing her voice caused me to burst into tears of fear, sadness, and apprehension of what I might find at the hospital. We arrived, parked our van, and quickly walked to the emergency room, unsure of what we might face there. Much to my surprise, we found an empty waiting room with not one single person there waiting that afternoon. The triage nurse took one look at Bennett and said, "He is having difficulty breathing," and I responded "Yes, I know. That is why we are here." The triage nurse then swiftly called back to the ER and immediately another nurse came running out to check Bennett, put masks on us, and help me wheel Bennett back.

We were whisked to a glass-enclosed room full of nurses dressed in blue isolation gowns with masks and face shields on. They slid the glass door shut, worked on Bennett to place an IV and then a respiratory BiPAP mask over his face for more oxygen and breathing support. I recall peering out the window at the crowd huddling together outside our room, as if I could hear the murmured discussion, "Will this be the next pediatric COVID-19 case to be reported to the D.C. Health Department?" I watched the entire scene unfold as if I had stepped out of my body and was floating above the room peering over all the activity. The nurses immediately drew blood to test Bennett for several different viruses, including COVID-19.

Bennett was eventually stabilized with acceptable vitals and was being cared for meticulously, so I was able to finally take a deep breath while I stood in the isolation room watching the hustle and bustle all around me. The medical professionals moved around the room like a well-oiled machine. Each staff person knew their role and responsibility in this crisis situation, and I stood in awe of them. They were very kind to me, answering my questions, and eventually the room emptied, as if they were theater performers exiting stage right. Bennett and I were left alone in the isolation room for more than four hours waiting for the virus test results. At times he fell asleep. Other times his big blue eyes looked around, over the large BiPAP mask, wondering where in the world he was. Eventually an excited nurse came in to report that he was negative for COVID, yet he had human metapneumovirus, a common virus like RSV. We were immediately admitted into the Pediatric Intensive Care Unit (PICU), and he could expect to be hospitalized four to five days as he recovered from it. I was relieved yet jolted that we were heading to the ICU, a place we had somehow avoided at this hospital until now. That day in the Children's National Hospital emergency room was a very surreal experience, considering it was the first week of the COVID-19 lockdown. In that moment we knew almost nothing about the virus, this invisible enemy. All we knew was that a mountain of uncertainty lay ahead for Bennett, our country, and our world.

Bennett was wheeled up to the PICU and settled into a bed surrounded by curtains in a large room that held at least eight beds, with a nursing station in the middle. There was no privacy at all, and no place for parents to sit other than small padded wooden chairs along the wall. I looked around, trying to quickly adapt to these new surroundings, familiar medical smells and sounds filling my sensory system. It was around midnight by that time, and I recall thinking, "I will need to find the restroom and vending machine. I am starving."

The body does have a way of adapting to new surroundings astonishingly quickly and I grew quite fond of one nurse immediately: another Nurse Ashley. This Ashley was blond and from outside of Baltimore, unlike our NICU Nurse Ashley who had been brunette and from North Carolina. As far as we were concerned, both nurses were angels sent from God. Blond Ashley immediately could tell that Bennett was very aware of his surroundings even though he could not physically tell us how he was feeling, what was hurting, or ask us to leave him alone when he was annoyed. My trust in her was rooted as we were settling into the PICU because she started talking directly to Bennett (looking into his eyes and rubbing his thick head of hair), immediately observing that he did not like the BiPAP mask. In fact, she wanted to get him transitioned off the BiPAP as quickly as possible because she suspected it was blowing too much air into his lungs. That first night confirmed her suspicions. Bennett coughed constantly throughout the night, unable to get comfortable to sleep. That was the first night I ever attempted to sleep in a small wooden chair, and the attempt was futile. I got no sleep because Bennett's cyclical coughing and vomiting encompassed each hour of the night, and I was wrestling with a mounting fear that this virus might morph into a life-threatening pneumonia. We had traveled that road nearly thirteen years before this, and it was difficult to push through those feelings of great fear and dread.

Travis came to the hospital the following day to take a "shift" and I went home to try to sleep after a nonexistent night's sleep in the small wooden hospital chair. This was the first week of the nationwide COVID-19 lockdown and yet our dear friend Julie, a Marine, mother of six children and naval doctor's wife, had insisted on taking our two younger kids hiking for the day. We had no other childcare option because all other family members were locked down in fear, so after Julie insisted on taking them, we agreed. It was a gift that Travis could be with Bennett, and I could get some sleep at home. Julie's small gesture meant the world to us because I needed sleep to boost my immune system and attempt to stay healthy myself. The world was shutting down by the minute, and it felt like an evil viral enemy lurked around every corner.

After a short nap, shower, and eating some food delivered by another dear friend, Moira, I wanted to return to the hospital that evening to see how Bennett was progressing. Travis had texted me that he was stable, but my mama bear instinct was telling me I had to see him with my own two eyes to evaluate whether he was improving or deteriorating. At that time, Children's National Hospital of D.C. had implemented COVID restrictions, but two parents were allowed to be with their child. In the PICU I saw that Bennett had improved slightly, but we were not close to leaving the PICU yet.

Travis kissed us goodbye and headed back to Julie's house to pick up our younger two children. He was planning to take them home to enjoy Moira's food and attempt a "normal" bedtime routine. As I stood in the PICU listening to the familiar sounds of beeping pumps, monitor alarms, and crying kids, all while inhaling the scents of fresh plastic tubing, alcohol swabs, and baby wipes, I could not believe we were trapped in the PICU amidst the beginning of a global pandemic. My eyes then gazed on the small wooden chair staring back at me, and I did not know whether I could wrestle with it again that night.

Bennett's breathing was slightly improved. They had removed the BiPAP machine, thanks to blond Nurse Ashley, and he was on a high-flow nasal cannula, allowing him to rest more peacefully. I sat down in the brown chair, attempted to scroll through my phone as the clock crept toward midnight, but was jolted by hunger pangs and decided to seek out food. As I headed out, the nurse told me that there was a parents' "sleep room" that I was welcome to check out. It included reclining chairs that parents could stretch out in. In the snack store I bought a packaged salad and bottled water, and then peeked into the "sleep room."

It took a few moments for my eyes to adjust to the darkness, but seeing the mounds of blankets covering bodies in recliners scattered throughout the large room, I took a mental note that I would come here if, and only if, I was completely desperate for sleep. After returning to Bennett's side, fixing his iPad's position and giving him a kiss goodnight, I sat in the small wooden chair, positioning a pillow between my head and the wall. I tossed and turned for what felt like hours, and eventually I caved. I told the PICU night charge nurse that I would be in the "sleep room" for a couple of hours and to come get me if they needed me. She smiled and nodded, agreeing that I needed some real rest.

Walking into a dark room filled with complete strangers, intending to fall asleep, is definitely not something I would encourage most people to do. Most certainly I would cringe at the thought of my children doing so. *Is this even safe?* I wondered. And yet as I walked in I said a prayer, asking God to protect me and Bennett, and asked Him to please give me some rest. I had carried with me a blanket and pillow our nurse had given me, so after finding a chair that was somewhat isolated I attempted to get comfortable in the sterile pleather recliner and eventually passed out for a few hours, surrounded by the mysterious bodies under mounds of blankets. Every now and then I heard the door quietly open, and a parent would either be walking out or walking in. In my sleep-deprived fog, I would reposition and drift back off to sleep. It was a very surreal experience that brought to my consciousness, once again, the deep humanity that exists among parents of critically ill children, the basic needs held by all people, and the fact that we are all more alike than different. Sleep heals, and we were all in need of some healing.

Bennett was discharged five days later after his lungs slowly improved, and his smiles, giggles, and "pep" came back. He had fought and beaten another virus, and for that we celebrated our strong young lad. We had watched the hospital TV around the clock as news of COVID-19 continued to evolve like a bad science-fiction movie, and were quickly realizing that although the world around us seemed to be hunkering down, bolting the doors, and preparing for impact, Children's National Hospital was eerily calm and quiet, nurses were being sent home because there were not enough patients to care for, all elective surgeries having come to a screeching halt; and things felt oddly "normal" as we gathered our belongings to head home and start living out this "new normal" which pandemic life was introducing to us all.

Bennett's school experience during COVID-19

After a few weeks at home, Bennett was back to full strength and he clearly enjoyed watching the videos that his beloved teacher, Ms. Cathy, had made for him and his class on her newly-created YouTube channel. Bennett smiled and giggled his deep belly laugh as Ms. Cathy sang morning songs, had circle time, read books, and even dressed up in costumes based on the theme of the day. Ms. Cathy made COVID-19 homeschooling a delight and thrill for our whole family in the spring of 2020.

Much to our dismay, one day in April 2020 we received news that a younger student at Bennett's school had passed away suddenly. She was very young, quite petite, and had a huge, beautiful smile—an angel. We did not know whether it was a seizure, stroke, pneumonia, and/or COVID-19-related, but her family desperately needed financial support to be able to release and prepare her body, hold a memorial at a local funeral home, and bury her. We were shaken with each update we received from the school, and in a matter of three days a small group of teachers, staff, and parents contributed more than $2500 for this mother during her time of great loss. Although it was disappointing that our large public-school system told us they had no benevolent funds to assist with such a request, Bennett's school community is small but mighty. This was yet another example of the beautiful and generous hearts there. Our school community is like *The Little Engine That Could,* and we take care of each other with the internal voice of "I think I can, I think I can" always in the heads of many of us. Our time, resources and energy are spread thin, but we always prove that nothing is impossible.

Communication between the angel's mother and concerned parents was strained because of language differences, but thank God we had Ms. Cece, our school sanitation officer, step in and translate via text all the visitation, memorial, and burial details. The night of the memorial came, and after checking in with school administrators and other parents, I realized that no one was able to attend the service. I deeply wanted to be there to honor this little angel, whom I believed was now in heaven, so I told my husband where I was headed that dark spring night. He asked me to please be careful. The older funeral home was nestled behind a busy intersection of a thoroughfare that leads straight into D.C. I parked my minivan and walked in, nodding at all the strangers' faces, trying to figure out where the child's mother was so that I could pay my respects to her.

In the funeral home's viewing room with its bright red carpet and golden fixtures, I saw adults and children standing around crying, and then my eyes darted to the angel lying in a small coffin. The sight of her took my breath away. She was dressed in the most beautiful white dress, her long flowing hair arranged perfectly, a rosary laced between her fingertips. I attempted to chat with her kind grandmother as tears rolled down her face. Then suddenly the angel's mother appeared. We embraced, I started to cry with her, and she led me up to the child's body. We cried together as I asked questions about her daughter, with sweet Cece next to me, translating, and before I knew it, the grieving mother stepped away to talk to a guest and I was left alone standing at the casket. I stood there stunned and sober, prayed and cried over her, and then softly stepped away.

I did not know this family or a single person in the packed funeral home besides Cece. Social distancing and masks had not really been implemented yet, so we were huddled together—I, the stranger in this tightly-knit group. And yet I did feel I knew them. This beautiful mother could have been myself at one of the many life-threatening times over Bennett's twelve years, and I know I will most likely be in her shoes one day. I might one day be greeting guests as they say goodbye to my child, me trying to hold back the tears, trying to put on a face of strength while I am dying inside.

We caregivers know daily challenges and hurdles, and yet what we really know is the beauty that comes with loving and serving a human being who can do nothing for themselves. They give us so much with their smiles, the sparkle in their eyes, or their deep sighs of contentment. Watching this angel's young cousins weep at her casket broke me in a way that I will never mend from. Children especially see the good in most people, regardless of education, class, ability, or wealth. Children are always willing to give the benefit of the doubt, and they try to bring a smile, or look for what is good, when hard is all around. Watching a child weep with grief is so unsettling because it is not the way this world is "supposed to be," and yet it is the reality that far too many know. That night at the funeral home I will never forget. I was humbled to be there. Celebrating the life of a precious child of God, gone too soon, was a gift to witness. She had a family and community that knew her and loved her, and for that I was very grateful.

After saying goodbye to the angel's mom, I walked back out to our minivan as the gravity of the moment hit me like a ton of bricks. That child's life meant something. She mattered. She had nothing to "give" to society, and yet her small hands and teeny-tiny fingers had been stroked by her mother's hands, her family members had held her, fed her, and/or comforted her, and for that their lives had been changed for the better. I know this to be true because I saw it in their eyes. I have watched the ways that Bennett's life has positively impacted the lives of those around us in profound ways. Sometimes that has left me shaking my head, saying to myself, "Only God. Only God could use something so very hard, exhausting, sad, and grueling, to bring more love, more patience, and more compassion to the world." When the entire world shut down in the spring of 2020, we all watched the case and death numbers tick up by the second on news programs, uncertainty and fear rippling across households and cities. It felt as though we were characters in a sci-fi motion picture as we watched the experts speak daily at COVID-19 press conferences, weighing the risks of going to the grocery store down the street. We locked down, watched as our county took rims off local park basketball backboards and taped off playgrounds with yellow police tape, all the while trying to keep calm as we attempted to explain these unprecedented actions to our elementary-school-aged kids. They looked up at us with huge bulging eyeballs each day, seeking answers about this changing world, and we tried our best to be steady, measured, and not panic. The wise words of my grandmother Mimi rang in my heart. I remembered her calmly speaking over me while attempting to teach me to float on my back in the waters of a public pool in Florida: "Whatever you do, do not panic."

We sat with our parents, socially distanced in yards and on porches, not hugging but longing to be near them and wanting to do all we could to keep them safe (this was months before the vaccines began to be administered). As the summer of 2020 progressed, we did more outdoor activities, traveled to see family, and paid close attention to the science and data rising to the surface above the divisive politics. We followed all the data very closely, using our own brains to make calculations and apply common sense while thinking critically. This virus was affecting every aspect of our family's life as well as our extended family members' small businesses, the lives of friends who worked on the front lines in hospitals, and other friends who were laid off as the global economy was in a free fall. Through it all we were committed to gathering information independently and objectively.

The virus was clearly serious, deadly, and spread quickly in certain circumstances, but we soon calculated that the death rate was actually much lower than experts had initially anticipated. An encouraging deduction was that the risk to younger, healthy people was quite low. As a result, educational and pediatric specialists in Europe and other parts of the world began encouraging schools to open in the fall of 2020, allowing kids to attend to continue their educational and social-emotional development. It was our hope that our school system would follow suit.

Unfortunately Bennett had to have the metal plates in his two hips removed in June of 2020. The metal plates had been placed in his double hip surgery back in 2017 and one plate was causing infection. COVID restrictions limited only one parent to be with him for this procedure, so Travis took him and I waited for them in the parking lot of the Chick-Fil-A closest to the hospital. It was a nerve-wracking time for us as the COVID precautions felt extreme, and the last time his hips were opened up, we spent six months recovering to fight infection and complications.

As Bennett was being wheeled back to surgery the anesthesiologist stopped Travis in the hall and said, "Are you Bennett's dad?" He was surprised to be recognized and said, "Yes, I sure am. Do we know you?" She replied that she had been an NICU fellow at Georgetown back in 2007 and she had never forgotten Bennett or his case. She would be working his case that day and she promised to take good care of him in the operating room. When Travis texted me this update I was instantly calmed and felt that once again, God had sent us an angel right when we needed it.

Bennett healed well from the metal plate extraction surgery and we were extremely grateful that he did not have any complications. Yet as the summer of 2020 neared an end, it became extremely clear to us that politics was now superseding the science and data regarding any change for in-person learning for him that fall. Our local elected officials had been burned by the local private schools which rolled out CDC-compliant, concrete plans to open for in-person learning in the fall. These private schools had lawyered up when our county initially refused to allow them to open, and the tension surrounding education was thick. Parents were fighting and virtue-signaling all over social media, fearmongering was rampant, and emotional manipulation was at its best. We live in an extremely educated and sophisticated county, and yet many refused to look to countries in Europe which had opened for in-person learning with proven success.

In February 2021, a large group of parents came together in support of re-opening the schools, standing with signs outside the county's educational administrative offices. By this point, in the US a large number of public-school systems across the country had opened for in-person learning as studies being released showed devastating consequences to the mental, social, and developmental growth of children. It was the coldest day of the year, but we all stood out there in the frigid whipping wind to stand up for our children's right to a safe in-person education. We all knew it was possible, because it had been proven possible by the local private schools and public-school systems across the world.

As I walked past a gentleman about sixty-five years old who was chatting with another participant, I heard him say, "I have never really stood up for any cause in my life. But this cause just felt like it was worth fighting for." I smiled as I walked by and appreciated his sentiments. This was a cause worth fighting for.

Bennett spent nearly fifty weeks sitting in our house during COVID-19 either in our kitchen, in his bed, or in our van when we took him out for drives. A few times we went out for walks, but he is very temperature-sensitive, so very cold or very hot days would make him as mad as a hornet. The state of Maryland's governor, Larry Hogan, finally came out in February of 2021 demanding that all counties in the state of Maryland present to him their plan to reopen for hybrid instruction no later than March 1, 2021. Bennett's school was one of the first schools penciled in to offer students in-person learning, and we had filled out the survey to indicate that we wanted him to attend. As March 1 approached, I did have conflicting feelings, mainly because I had worked alongside others tirelessly over the past six months to get to this day where we had an option. On the other hand, I was concerned that perhaps I was putting him at risk of getting the virus—something that we had somehow dodged thus far. After meeting with our beloved pediatrician, he talked through a risk assessment with us, listened to our situation, and gave us the green light while telling us, "Bennett, go be a trailblazer!"

When the short yellow school bus pulled up to our house on the rainy morning of March 1, 2021, it was surreal and wonderful. Bennett had his mask on, the bus driver and attendant were masked, and they seemed genuinely happy to see him after nearly a year. Overall, it was a morning full of positivity, joy, and hope. My gut kept telling me that we had to start somewhere to get kids back in public school, and this felt like more than a win. It felt like a triumph. Many parents throughout our large county saw pictures of Bennett and read news articles mentioning his journey, and we got nothing but positive and encouraging feedback. I had fully prepared myself for the negative Nellies of the world, but on March 1, 2021, there was nothing but relief, tears, and love for a little boy in a wheelchair who could not walk or talk but giggled the entire bus ride to school. The school bus and his school happen to be two of his favorite places and he remained healthy and happy on through June when the school year concluded. Our county was in last place in the entire nation to return to in-person learning, and yet Bennett was one of the first to lead the way back. For that we will always be grateful.

CHAPTER 20

Gratitude Versus Fear

"Pain and suffering have come into your life,
but remember: Pain, sorrow, suffering are
but the kiss of Jesus—a sign that you have come
so close to Him that He can kiss you."
— Mother Teresa

WE DO NOT KNOW why our son survived his traumatic birth when so many other children do not. We do not have the answer to the universally difficult question, "Why does a good God let bad things happen?" We know that many parents of children with severe disabilities do not have family, friends, or community support like we have had along Bennett's journey. Large numbers of families suffer with financial, emotional, physical, and mental health crises, along with divorce rates of well over 80 percent, when caring for a child with disabilities. Every day we attempt to focus on what we have, not on all that we do not have—focusing on the good that we have been given.

In no way are we insinuating we have been given a Pollyanna-like reality while other families face the depth of heartache, pain, and struggle that accompanies around-the-clock care of loved ones with disabilities. We stand right along with all the parents who are caring for a loved one. We feel their pain and we acknowledge the endless days of waking up to bathe, diaper, change clothes, feed, re-position, wipe drool, calm tears or fits, drive to doctor appointments, spend hours on the phone with doctors/insurance/state benefits offices, and fill out the never-ending paperwork. We stand with you and we see you. Every minute of every day.

We stand with you when you get the startled look from a stranger who does not know how to greet you as you walk into a store pushing your child in a wheelchair. We stand with you when the waiter barely comes to your restaurant table because they find it too uncomfortable that your child is so loud and "distracting." We stand with you when you somehow get your family plopped onto the beach to enjoy the sand in your toes, and strangers all around give you uncomfortable glances that make you feel as if your loud or "imperfect" kid is ruining *their* perfect day in the sand. And we stand with you when you are trying to keep your disabled child happy in the doctor's waiting room (after you have already been there forty-five minutes) and you are then told the doctor is still running at least another hour behind.

We do not think we are in any way special or more deserving than other families who have suffered in similar or different ways. In fact, we are so *not special, not elite*, and *not entitled* that we are constantly surprised when life with Bennett has opened doors and provided opportunities that felt "special." It is an honor to stand on a stage and give a talk about Bennett's life, just as it was an honor to get handed a game ball at a Washington Nationals baseball game (the autumn that they won the World Series) or play games on the lawn of the White House for the Easter Egg Roll. We are not more special or more deserving than anyone else. For some reason, the world has made a place for Bennett Speck at the table. Strangers long to be near him, and it truly feels as if we get to live with our own little version of a fictional character who warmed the hearts of millions just a few decades ago, Forrest Gump: "Life is like a box of chocolates. You never know what you're gonna get." We had no idea what we were going to get, and yet life with Bennett is sweeter by the day.

Not long after Bennett's birth we were told by close friends, who had the best of intentions, "We are so sorry this happened. You guys did not deserve this." We appreciated their sincerity and concern, yet those statements have always stuck with me and quite frankly made me uncomfortable. This is because, in my opinion, no one "deserves" to watch their baby almost bleed to death, be told your baby was going to die, mentally prepare for a newborn's funeral, unexpectedly have your baby live with severe disabilities and be 100 percent dependent on you for the remainder of their life. That is not how God works, sending down suffering on those who "deserve it." We live in a broken and complex world and have ever since sin entered the world. But we do believe and trust in the sovereignty of God, not because it sounds good and gives you warm fuzzies like rainbows or unicorns, but because we have experienced His faithfulness day in and day out, in both the uneventful and the miserably agonizing days.

We have had more difficult days than we could ever count. Yet in the quiet moments of that desolate isolation, there has always been a deep sense that we are not alone. We may feel as if we are bobbing on a lifeboat in the middle of the ocean, yet we know we are not abandoned. We have looked up to those who had experienced similar circumstances, like Mike and Diane Cope, Gene and Ruth Stallings, Lon and Brenda Solomon, and Jim and Jill Kelly. Each of these couples with children with disabilities has lived through extreme challenges watching their children suffer (each chronicled in their own books), felt the stress on all family members, and yet celebrate the blessing that these precious little souls were here on their earth.

"We rejoice in our sufferings, knowing that suffering produces endurance, and endurance produces character, and character produces hope." — Romans 5:3-4

Our journey with Bennett has been a roller coaster from day one, and that ride only continues. Some days the hills and dips feel less extreme; other times it feels as if we are heading up a huge hill—click-click-click—knowing that a free fall is imminent. In fact, as I previously mentioned, in addition to being responsible for entertaining, soothing him, and caring for him every waking minute of his day for his entire life, keeping him safe and free from harm is another concern that is on our minds every minute of every day. *Is the guardrail up on his hospital bed in his room so that he does not tumble to the ground? Has he been re-positioned enough today so that he does not get any bed sores? He is sleeping extra late today; are we sure that he did not aspirate his overnight feed? Is he breathing? Are his eyes tracking? As I roll him down our steep driveway to go on a walk, what if I trip or faint and he rolls into the street into oncoming busy traffic?*

Travis and I enjoy being outside, and therefore we get our kids outside as much as we can. Sometimes they like it, other times they complain, but we get pretty stir-crazy if we are inside for too long, so they have come to accept this reality, Bennett included. A positive aspect of our area is that there are parks all around us, with paths and green space abounding. Back when Bennett was in a jogging stroller we could "off road" and do more trails, but after he transitioned to a wheelchair, we became limited to paved paths and roads. Bennett loves to look up at the green tree leaves above him. He watches the light reflections as they change, and the cool breeze against his face often has him dozing off into a relaxed catnap.

Rock Creek Park is a national park in Washington, D.C., spanning two thousand acres, and is known for its expansive greenspace amidst the city. Travis and I spent many days walking together along the Rock Creek Park paths years before we had children, so now that we have children it is a "full circle" joy for us to explore the many paths and trails there. During the COVID lockdowns, the District of Columbia decided to not allow cars on the weekends on the street that runs through the middle of the park. As a result, people on foot, bikes, and scooters are welcome to use the road as a path, all in an effort to allow for outdoor recreation with social distancing and safety. It worked out well for our family as our younger two kids can walk along the bumpy path, climb rocks, and ascend trails up along the hills that line the roads while Bennett is pushed along the smooth street or path.

Bennett's auditory senses have always been very strong, so we love for him to hear the rushing rapids of the Rock Creek amidst the birds chirping and the ker-plunk of rocks being skipped into the creek by his brother. In our efforts to include him, embrace his limitations, and give him as many experiences as we possibly can, we will attempt to give him the best views on the banks of the creek. While trying to enjoy the refreshing moment soaking up the beautiful scenery, watching his eyes delight in the light's reflection off the leaves and rocks, I still battle the thoughts of *Hold on tight to the wheelchair. Whatever you do, don't let go. Watch out for anyone passing by who could accidentally make his wheelchair plummet down the bank into the creek.* I fully recognize that this might sound crazy or irrational, but it is our reality.

In fact, a fear that can overtake me and cause me to shudder in panic is when we cross over bridges spanning a large body of water, like the Chesapeake Bay Bridge. The Bay Bridge was the world's longest continuous over-water steel structure when it opened in 1952. The bridge is more than four miles long and connects Maryland's eastern shore with its urban western shore, a path we travel regularly during the summer months. *What if this car plummets into the water? We could not get Bennett out of his chair and the car.* It is a nightmare that has jarred me awake from a deep sleep on multiple occasions. And if you know me at all, you know how deeply and soundly I sleep. I once fell asleep in a small boat rowing across a creek in Honduras. True story. Very few things wake me up or prevent me from sleeping, but the what-ifs of keeping Bennett safe do haunt me. And yet, after a few deep breaths and some centering into what I know to be true, scriptures like this, etched into my heart and soul, are what keep me from living in a constant state of fear or panic:

> "Fear not, for I am with you. Be not dismayed, for I *am* your God. I will strengthen you, Yes, I will help you, I will uphold you with My righteous right hand." — Isaiah 41:10

We fully recognize that many unknowns still lie ahead for our family. We know that Bennett will most likely face medical challenges in the future as his body grows and matures, plus we have no idea of what his life expectancy will be. There will most likely be struggles in the future not only for Bennett but for his parents and even his siblings. None of us know what the future holds, yet our experiences have taught us that striving for peace far outweighs a life full of fear or anxiety amidst uncertainty. Trusting in God, surrendering our plans, and being willing to adapt to the circumstances that rise up to meet us, are the actions that allow us to seek true peace in the arms of hope.

We live a very full life, daily trying to celebrate the "wins" (he didn't cry or throw up today!) and push through the "defeats" (he needs another surgery or is severely constipated). Bennett is now a young man full of personality and joy, and his life really is a gift. His life is a gift. This is not something we say to sound cliché, or to tie a nice bow on a package wrapped with torn paper with pieces of tape barely holding it together.

Every time we walk past Bennett sitting in his wheelchair, usually at the end of our kitchen island (his favorite spot), he smiles at us. If we lie in his bed with him kissing his cheeks, we get a deep belly laugh and his eyes light up with joy. When he is lying in his bed and we swing his legs off the bed, sit him up straight, and hold him close for a hug, he always gives us a long, contented sigh. Bennett usually then looks around hurriedly until he sees who is hugging him and gives us a big smile. It's almost as if he is thinking, "Boy, did I need that hug. I love you." We are grateful for every hug we get from him and we treasure each long sigh that he exhales. His presence, smiles, and giggles fill our house and can make a "bad" or "sad" day brighter. Sunnier days are a gift from this child who cannot say a single word.

Bennett's life is a gift because knowing him and caring for him has changed us in every respect. Having Bennett Mitchell Speck has given us a perspective on life that we would never have had if we had lived a "typical" life of marriage, two-and-a-half kids, and a white picket fence. There is nothing wrong with that life. Heck, *we* wanted that life, and many people live very full and purposeful lives with "typical" circumstances. Neither is right or wrong; we are all given the hand we are dealt. The beauty is, the hand *we* were dealt is so radically different than anything we could have ever imagined in our wildest dreams that we were faced with an implicit decision much earlier in life than most, well before we each turned thirty years old.

The unspoken question being thrown in our faces at the age of twenty-nine was: Will this "hand" completely devastate us, causing unrecoverable devastation, bitterness, and sorrow, or were we going to allow this "hand" to mature us and bless us? To teach us, to refine us, to redefine us, to redeem us? To break us down and then build us up into the people we were truly meant to be? When you fold back all the distractions, isn't that what life is? Daily we are given choices as to how we will respond to the events which have unfolded. The only thing that we can control is how we respond to what life throws at us.

Some days we are brave and respond positively with energy and focus. Other days we can barely lift our heads off our pillows to face the nightmare that is the current reality. Both responses are completely warranted, and we have experienced each of them, plus nearly every emotion on the spectrum. During our most difficult seasons of suffering, it has been our experience that grace for ourselves and those we love dearly is crucial for walking through the most difficult of days. Grace is the key to allowing ourselves, and those closest to us, to cope with the current circumstances in whichever way they deem appropriate for that moment. No judgement. No criticism. Only grace.

"I do not at all understand the mystery of grace—only that it meets us where we are but does not leave us where it found us." — Anne Lamott

If Bennett had not lived in those first days following ECMO in September 2007, we hope that we would have recovered from the devastating loss of our firstborn. We hope that we would have stayed married (over 80 percent of marriages that have buried a child end in divorce). We hope that we would have kept clinging to our faith. We hope that we would have stayed in Christian community with those who loved us. We hope that we would not have turned to darkness, despair, or hopelessness. But we thank God every single day that Bennett did live, and we simply ask God daily for more wisdom, more understanding, and more strength to care for Bennett with the dignity and love that he deserves. It is hard? Yes. It is humbling? Yes. Does it strip us of our own pride? Yes. Is it easy? Not at all.

Caring for Bennett's every need can feel overwhelming and unrelenting, yet we have a rewarding and meaningful life. All these feelings can exist together in harmony under one roof. We know this because it reflects our life. Ensuring he has his medications, his formula, a clean bed, placing each leg in his pants, placing his shirts over his head of thick hair, brushing his teeth, combing his hair, finding a clean bib to catch his drool, and ensuring he has his favorite toys within reach are all tasks that occur every single day, usually multiple times a day. That is in addition to soccer and baseball practices, school activities, friend gatherings, hosting sleepovers, and traveling to see family near and far. It is bonkers, and it is beautiful. Bennett continues to give us all the perspective we will ever need. Our perspective is broadened, our "wins" are not typical, and we are most grateful for the dull days when everyone is healthy, rested, safe, and at peace.

CHAPTER 21
Digging Into Faith

*"Most people feel best about themselves when they
give their best to something greater than themselves."*
— John Maxwell

FAITH HAS BEEN a part of our lives and our marriage from the very beginning. We were both born into families in which following Christ was a priority and God's love was spoken about regularly. We were raised in communities of faith that were not perfect, but we experienced the transforming beauty of Christian community while eating casseroles at church potlucks, playing hide-and-seek in our church buildings, attending church camp during a week of the summer, and singing *a capella* hymns at the tops of our lungs. We felt the warm hugs of older parishioners of our congregations and our value system was greatly influenced by the love faith communities poured into us.

I mentioned that the night that my water broke on August 19, 2007, right before we went to the hospital to deliver Bennett, the daily scriptures in the *One Year Bible* I was reading were quite startling. As I am a firm believer that nothing is a coincidence, when I look back to these passages I see that they might have been preparing my heart for the journey that we were about to embark upon with Bennett.

In the New International Version (NIV) of the *One Year Bible* that I was reading, there was a passage from both the Old Testament and a passage from the New Testament for each day of the year. Ironically, the Old Testament passage that day included infamous words from Esther 4:14: "And who knows but that you have come to this position for such a time as this?" As I read ahead to the next day's passage for August 20, the passages were from Esther 8:1-10:3, in which Esther's leadership saved her people, the Jews, from oppression and death. This just so happens to be my favorite story in the Bible. I have always admired the bravery, principled leadership, and strength that Esther showed in the face of great risk and danger to her own life. Esther might have been afraid, deep down; but she did not show fear, she trusted God, and she led with integrity. After finishing that day's scriptures late that night, well past midnight, I had a deep restlessness within me. I tossed and turned, trying to sleep, but I simply could not, so I read ahead to the passage for August 21, which began with Job 1:1.

As I lay there reading in the dark of night, I was reminded that Job lost all at once his entire material wealth—his oxen, sheep, and camels all perished, along with all his working staff. Following the news of these great economic losses, Job is notified that his children were all killed while feasting together at the oldest brother's house. Instead of cursing God and dropping his faith like a hot coal, Job tore his robe, shaved his head, and cried out, "Naked I came from my mother's womb, and naked I will depart. The Lord gave, the Lord has taken away; may the name of the Lord be praised."

In no way do I think that I am like Esther or that we have suffered in ways that are comparable to Job. But both these examples of faith inspire me, and they were highlighted for me hours before Bennett was born. I will never see that as a coincidence. I will say that during our almost fifteen years of caring for Bennett, it has felt at times that the luxuries, distractions, conveniences, identities, stature, and material values have been taken from us. Certain things we might have previously longed for or valued were simply not an option. We spent months sitting in hospital rooms with sick children, so we did not have the time, energy, or money to host a dinner party, try out a new recipe, or purchase the car, house, or wardrobe that we longed for. Any of our previous thirty-year-old desires were not compatible with the exhausting list of tasks that encompassed our daily life with Bennett.

At some point I recall realizing that I had missed the tutorial on "How to host a cozy dinner party." You know, the ones where there are melt-in-your-mouth appetizers, food-blogger-approved main dishes, and delicious desserts to top off the meal, all paired with the most perfect wine for each course. Unfortunately, I do not remember much of my thirties. It feels as though I lost a decade of my life in the sense that my thirties are nothing but a blur. I know we had three kids, spent a lot of time changing diapers, were in and out of the hospital, plus worked multiple jobs while attempting to feed and grow little humans to keep them as safe and healthy as possible.

With my whole heart I can say that I am grateful for the refining that has taken place in our hearts while walking along this journey. Being Bennett's parents has made us more compassionate. Our hearts are more aware of the pain in this world, and our eyes are more open to the suffering that presents in the lives of many, many people. Even in the lowest of low moments when I could not see that any good could come from either Bennett's suffering or our excruciating pain, I knew that God was with us. I never questioned His existence or His power. I knew that God could and would either open our eyes to His plan or show us His plan to work for good. I know that He is a loving God who never abandons those who love Him. I know that He is a God who stays close to the brokenhearted.

"The Lord is close to the brokenhearted and saves those who are crushed in spirit." — Psalms 34:18

And finally, I know that a life hoping for the promises of heaven and trusting and leaning on Him each minute of each day was the only life in which my soul could find true contentment. The trendy self-help slogans of, "You do you," or "Trust the universe" were not going to get us through the turbulent trials we have faced. You see, if there was no God, and this was all happening because "the universe" had willed it to happen, I do not believe that I would have had the strength, peace, and fortitude to function in the first three years of Bennett's life. The days of hospitalizations, constant physical therapy, feeding, calming, screaming, nonstop gastrointestinal issues, and vomiting required an endless amount of steady determination. I knew that we had witnessed a miracle when God saved Bennett in the NICU just forty-eight hours following his removal from the ECMO heart-lung bypass machine. Few people can say that they witnessed a miracle, but there is no doubt that we did. No medical professional could explain to us why Bennett survived coming off ECMO.

In a similar way, in the Book of John, chapter 6, Jesus's disciples had witnessed the miracle of Jesus feeding more than five thousand people after beginning with a mere five loaves of bread and two fish. Yet even after witnessing this logically impossible miracle, some of Jesus's followers abandoned Him and stopped following Him. After seeing them walk away, Jesus immediately asked His twelve disciples if they wanted to leave Him too. He had just performed a jaw-dropping miracle with no explanation, and yet some were unimpressed and went on their merry way.

The Lord could have asked Travis and me if we "wanted to leave Him" as well in our lowest moments of getting Bennett's MRI results and learning of his cerebral palsy diagnosis. As God watched us wrestle with our deep grief and pain He might have wondered, "I just saved your son from the grip of death, and yet with this devastating diagnosis, are you now going to leave Me?" Thanks to the prayers of saints and grace pouring over us during that time, our hearts never once considered turning away from our faith. We did not understand why any of these unexplainable disasters were happening to our son's newborn body, nor why God was allowing our son to suffer in such horrific ways. There was no cliché or Bible verse to wrap it up all neatly with a bow. But abandoning our faith or turning away from trusting God was honestly never even discussed. We were not taking our hearts elsewhere.

"Simon Peter answered him, 'Lord, to whom shall we go? You have the words of eternal life.'" — John 6:68

As a parent of a disabled child, mottos like "Be true to yourself" or "Follow your truth" are empty self-help slogans and not at all helpful to me. There is no self-help mantra to pull you out of the hell that so many people experience in hospital rooms, medical waiting rooms, on the site of a tragic car accident, or in the quiet of one's home. If you have been in a place of deep grief, suffering, devastation, hopelessness, or despair, there is a God of the universe who knows you, who loves you, and who sits with you in the darkest moments of your life. He knows you because He created you, and He has great plans for your life. Nothing that the Lord creates is a mistake. As David wrote in a psalm:

"For You created my inmost being; You knit me together in my mother's womb." — Psalm 139:13

The mystery of God is real, and I have grown to find comfort in the mystery of His ways, not abandonment. The fact is, if I did not have the hope of one day being face-to-face with Jesus while I watch

Bennett run, jump, and talk in heaven, I would not be able to get out of bed each morning to care for anyone else, let alone myself. On the extra heavy days where hope seems distant, this scripture is especially encouraging:

"Let the morning bring me word of Your unfailing love, for I have put my trust in You. Show me the way I should go, for to You I entrust my life." — Psalm 143:8

The deep loneliness and isolation one can experience when wrestling with deep suffering or horrific circumstances of this world can feel like the weight of a wet buffalo on your back. We have felt the weight of hopelessness, despair, or thoughts such as "No one could ever understand how hard our life is." These are completely normal and human feelings to have, and we can relate on every level. And yet we were not created to attempt to shoulder the burdens of this broken world alone. We were created to be in relationship. Sometimes life includes relationships with others amidst our suffering, but sometimes we suffer alone or autonomously, with the only conversations occurring between our heart and God. In the moments when it seems as if hope is out of our grasp and/or God may feel distant, cling to the fact that we have a Creator, Father, and Savior who tells us these words of comfort:

"Come to me, all you who are weary and burdened, and I will give you rest. Take My yoke upon you and learn from Me, for I am gentle and humble in heart, and you will find rest for your souls." — Matthew 11:28-29

CHAPTER 22
Final Reflections

"He's not dead. He is still alive, and
while he is alive, he is mine."
— Paullina Simons

A S WE NEARED the end of writing this manuscript, our family of five was at a baseball game for Jackson. It was at a picturesque park in northern Maryland with rolling green hills, blooming azaleas, and a gentle breeze filling the spring night. Jackson played a great game, Reagan spent the evening doing cartwheels with friends under pine trees, with the sap from the trees covering her bare legs. As the game wound down, two little preschool girls walked up to Bennett's wheelchair as we were walking along the paved path behind the backstop. One girl's big brown eyes looked at us as she asked, "Is he even alive? Because he doesn't look alive." I smiled at them, their precious faces bewildered with honest curiosity. I replied with, "He is alive! In fact, he is very alive. He just cannot walk or talk like you, but he actually has a lot of things he likes." They smiled and skipped away, and I was moved by the simple conversation. Bennett is alive indeed. He is very alive. He is more alive and more aware of his world than we will ever know.

As a child who cannot speak, cannot tell us what hurts, cannot complain about a sibling, or tell us his favorite football team, Bennett's life has significantly impacted the lives of others, some of whom we do not even know, and changed the trajectory of their lives. When God spared Bennett's life in September 2007, this inspired Andy, a college friend of ours in medical school at the time, to pursue a neonatology specialization.

Regarding Andy's decision to go into neonatology, his wife, Amy, shared with us, "It's impossible to fully understand it unless you've been there, but it really gave both of us insight and perspective into what parents and families experience and the road they face. That kind of understanding is invaluable and makes such a huge difference to parents when NICU docs and staff can validate that what they are going through is life-altering, traumatic, and set apart. It's not a hospital stay, it's a full-on war, and it's an enormous mountain to overcome. That's the case with almost all NICU babies. And then there's ones like Bennett, whose cases are truly heartbreaking and infuriating because they so vividly illuminate how unfair life can be. But then you see those babies down the road and hear about what their lives mean to so many people, and you realize that God uses even the seriously tragic for good when we just let Him. Bennett helped solidify Andy's choice to pursue neonatology, and he's helped save hundreds of babies and touched so many families since that time. I can't tell you how often I run into someone who had Andy take care of their baby, and it's always the same—he was so caring, so comforting, so compassionate, and so funny, all when they needed exactly that. And we hear it from friends of friends and others. As you know, you have to be a special kind of person to work in the NICU, and sweet baby Bennett, you are a huge part of Andy being one of those special people."

In the summer of 2016, Travis was able to meet up with some college friends at the lake house of his friend, Darren. They had a wonderful weekend of catching up on life and he came away from the weekend encouraged after reconnecting with friends over fifteen years post-college. Darren soon after reached out to me asking for a few pictures of Bennett, because Darren had a close friend who was an artist, and he wanted to surprise Travis with something related to Bennett. I had no idea what he was planning, so I emailed over a few pictures and honestly completely forgot about the entire thing. A few months passed, and before we knew it, a large two-by-two-and-a-half-foot canvas appeared wrapped on our doorstep. Travis opened up the brown packaging and he stood stunned looking at a beautiful hand-painted canvas of me holding Bennett on the beach, and three strong horses peering down over us through the reeds in the sand.

The artist had heard that Travis's favorite Bible passage was in 2 Kings 6:8-23 when it says, "And Elisha prayed, 'Open his eyes, Lord, so that he may see.' So the Lord opened the eyes of the young man and he saw; and behold, the mountain was full of horses and chariots of fire all around Elisha." Travis had mentioned to Darren that he draws strength knowing that on days that feel particularly heavy, he can always rest assured that the Lord is sending him an army of angels to face any battle that day may bring. The artist had brought this passage to life through the gentle strokes of paint with his talented hand.

The talented artist included a card reading, "Just as the fiery armies of heaven were with Elisha, so we also walk in the ever-present shadow of the divine. The horses in this painting are a poignant reminder of the beauty of God's strength, majesty and gentleness. This reality of the unseen presence of God with us and His love for us is expressed in the steady presence of the Father, that powerful saving love of the Son, and the gentle nearness of the Holy Spirit . . ." We were blown away and continue to be each time we look at this wondrous piece of art that hangs in our dining room.

Speaking of blown away, we were equally blown away by a letter given to us telling us how Bennett had affected one woman's life. This woman in Florida had walked away from her Christian faith as a teenager, and by the age of twenty-one she had closed the book entirely on God, belief, faith, and prayer. She was a regular reader of her cousin's blog, and on August 22, 2007, a blog post entitled "Prayers Please" caught her attention. She got wrapped up reading about Bennett's daily fight for his life, and as he lay in the NICU knocking on death's door the night he was removed from ECMO, she asked her husband, a critical-care doctor, if there was any chance Bennett might survive. Her husband gave her a look that pretty much reduced her to tears.

The Florida woman stared at her computer, unable to see the words blurred through her tears. She later told us, "After several minutes, a voice from the distant past suddenly rose up in me, and I prayed. I prayed for the first time in years. I prayed and I didn't stop. I prayed for his lungs, I prayed like a faithful servant of God, I prayed and prayed for Bennett Mitchell Speck. I, and hundreds, possibly thousands, of people prayed for Bennett on that crucial night. The events that have unfolded since then have left me in a somewhat shocked and confused state. What happened inside me? What happened inside Bennett's lungs? Can science and medicine alone explain it? What does this mean for me? I was pretty much a non-believer, yet when it came down to it, I prayed. And if I prayed, then I must have some faith. This is something that has had my head spinning in the days since. I believe it is time to re-examine my closed book. I'm not sure where this journey will lead me, but I am sure that it is a [faith] journey that has begun because of a little baby boy that I have never met named Bennett." When Bennett did indeed survive coming off of ECMO and it appeared that he was going to live, she sent us another letter telling us, "[t]he night of September 6 was a turning point not only for your boy, but for me as well. Since I wrote that letter, I have been engaged in quite a few very passionate and deep discussions with several people about God, faith, and prayer. One of the most memorable discussions was with my husband. He was following Bennett's progress with me, and he was truly amazed at Bennett's ability to sustain his breathing when he went off ECMO. My husband deals with life and death every day and has done so for thirteen years without any belief in God; but this, this, made him shake his head and say to me, 'I don't know. I just don't know. Maybe this is something we should explore.' So right now we are in the process of trying to 'pick a church.' I'm not even really sure how you go about doing that, but we both decided that we want our two young boys to grow up with God in their lives."

Reading these letters from the Florida woman gave us a greater awareness that this circumstance in which we found ourselves had a much greater purpose than we could comprehend. We were stunned that our Creator was using the life of a baby boy bleeding to death in an NICU in Washington, D.C., to bring families to faith down in sunny south Florida. Equally powerful is the fact that an artist in Texas would take the hours out of his busy schedule to gift a complete stranger with a moving piece of art and a letter to encourage us along our journey. It is baffling, it is humbling, it is mysterious, and only the mystery of God could fully understand it.

Fast forward ten years to the summer of 2017 when Bennett's double hip surgery had occurred, multiple complications had resulted, and, desperate to "get away," we rented a small condo at a nearby beach for a week. One day while we were at the pool letting the littler two kids swim, we literally ran into one of our beloved NICU nurses, Adele, whom we had not seen in nearly ten years. We said hello, hugged, and realized that her family was staying right around the corner from us for the week as well. We could not believe what a small world it was. We chatted and planned to bring Bennett to her condo so she could see him. Unfortunately, the week got away from us and we did not get a chance to swing by to see Adele before we departed from the beach.

Not too long after our run-in with Adele at the pool, I read via her Facebook page that her health had taken a major turn for the worse and she had spent months hospitalized as she battled a mysterious illness. I kept up with her journey from afar, praying that her health would be fully restored, and with the speed of daily life, several years went by. As we began the process for writing this manuscript I reached out to Adele and a few other nurses to get any memories they might have of Bennett's birth experience. I knew that Bennett's case had been memorable, but I also knew that these nurses had seen a lot of sick babies come through to be cared for through the years.

I was surprised when Adele wrote back immediately, sharing, "You all are an inspiration and a family that I will always hold near and dear to my heart. I have called on your memory many times when I felt I was too tired or overwhelmed to continue fighting what feels like an endless medical battle."

The notion that the pain we lived out in front of a young, energetic, and healthy nurse while we sat in old pleather-lined gliders under the dimmed lights of the NICU, could give her strength as she faced her own giants in her very serious health battle is something that only God could have orchestrated. He brought us into each other's lives for a very specific purpose—one we do not fully understand, and yet we are eternally grateful. Adele provided us words of encouragement in some of our lowest moments, and through the mystery of God she was able to draw on her memories with us while she fought her own physical battles.

What is this "hope"?

"My joy is nonnegotiable." — Kathie Lee Gifford

For many reading our story, your life is most likely nothing like ours, and yet you may have experienced deep pain, or you know someone living amidst deep pain. When you watch a friend or loved one hurting, at times it can feel quite hopeless, and you might feel completely help-less. We can relate to both. We encourage you to show up for them in whatever way you can and walk with them in whatever way they allow you to do so.

In our life experiences since Bennett's birth, our eyes have been opened to the fact that many people we come in contact with are in desperate need of joy. Most people gladly welcome a smile and a genuine "Have a great day!" People usually respond with sincere appreciation when we take the time to smile and say "Thank you" when we grab our to-go order from our favorite local establishment's worker, or when our health tech comes to tidy up while we sit in a hospital room. I am always warmed and amazed at the response when we attempt to spread joy rather than negativity or complaints. The simple question of "How is your day going?" or "Wow, I love your nails!" can bring a look of surprise and then gratitude when we take the time to notice, acknowledge, and appreciate the people we come across on our daily paths. We all share the universal human need of being seen, and a little boy dependent on us for life has helped to open our eyes to this truth.

"Be kind, for everyone you meet is fighting a battle you know nothing about." — Author unknown

We were each twenty-nine years old when Bennett was born. We may never fully know what happened the day of Bennett's birth, nor why he suffered brain damage and will spend his life in a wheelchair or a bed. Some days the pain of his condition leaves us weeping through-out the day, and yet sometimes the sting is less painful.

We share our story of Bennett's birth and life with the world to encourage and uplift you regarding what you have faced, are facing, or will face in the future. We have stared death in the face, felt the devastation of a life-altering diagnosis, and have spent nearly a decade and a half bouncing from one crisis to another crisis. One universal fact is that we will all experience pain at some point in our lives.

"What brings us to tears will bring us to grace. Our pain is never wasted." — Bob Goff

Perhaps you already have great pain, or one day in the future great pain will appear out of nowhere. We wish it were not the case, but our experiences have taught us that pain is the universal condition. We encourage you to dig deep, cry out to the Creator of the universe, seek out wise and good people around you (they are there, we promise), surrender your pain, and hold tight to the hope that you are not alone in what you are experiencing. In each of our personal circumstances, there certainly is real, momentous, debilitating pain in our lives, and/ or in the lives of people all around us. The good news is that the story does not end there, and never will end with pain, because there is always hope in the heartache.

"I have told you these things, so that in Me you may have peace. In this world you will have trouble. But take heart! I have overcome the world." — John 16:33

In our house, our peace comes from holding on tight to the hope of what God holds for our future. We have a Savior: He made you, He loves you, and He is close to the brokenhearted. He is walking alongside you on your journey, in both your joys and your pain. If you do not know Him, He is a gentleman waiting for you to say His name. He made a sacrifice for us all by dying on the cross to wipe away the evil, pain, and sin from all the world. Because of His great love, He wants to have us all with Him in heaven for eternity—not because of anything we have done to deserve it, but because His love is so deep, so wide, so steadfast, and so faithful.

Chad Veach, a pastor in California, once said, "Hope is not an optimistic outlook or wishful thinking." For those of us who do not believe that we are here on earth for a random period of time, intersecting with things that "the universe" is throwing at us, we actually have a rock-solid understanding of what hope is. Hope is the confident expectation of what God has promised and its strength in His faithfulness. What has God promised? That we have the opportunity to one day meet Him face to face in heaven and live there for all eternity with Him, His Son, and all the saints that have gone before us. The thing our family looks most forward to is the day we get to run, walk, and talk with Bennett in heaven. What a glorious day that will be.

ACKNOWLEDGEMENTS

Thank you to our parents, siblings, and family members who have never left our sides. We know there is nothing you would not do for us or our children, and there is no way to express all the ways you have made our burdens lighter. We love you so much.

To the army of people who walked with us during Bennett's birth and the seventy days in the NICU, we can never properly thank you for your support. You carried us with your prayers and were truly the wind beneath our wings. Forgive us for anyone we may have forgotten, but we have deep gratitude to our steadfast and loyal families, Fairfax Church of Christ, Brentwood Hills Church of Christ, Stacie and Stuart, Erica and Matt, Laura and Brent, Colleen and Phil, Gretchen and Jeff, Robin and Jeremy, Margaret and Doug, Elizabeth and Brandon, Tafaney, Rachel, Kalli, Tiffany, Justin, Sarah and Kevin, Beth and J.P., Shanta and Ken, Ginger and Cody, Holly and Jonathan, Todd, Julia and Darren, Amanda and David, Ann and Darren, Amy and Andy, Yasmin, our co-workers at the NIH, and Winston, who showered us with gifts and support. Thank you to our ACU friends and acquaintances who prayed and contributed to gifts, and to the many friends and strangers around the world who cared enough to pray for a little boy in Washington, D.C. fighting for his life.

Thank you for checking the website for daily NICU updates and for sending us a "prayer page." Some of you sent us letters, pictures, and gifts that we still cherish to this day. Others dropped into the Georgetown NICU after driving or flying in from far away, just to hug us and be present in our pain. We will never be able to fully express our deep gratitude for all the ways you cared for us.

To the High Hopes community who welcomed a feisty eighteen-month-old into your pediatric therapy center, helped him take steps on the treadmill, and always had a boombox within reach to keep his attention, we cannot thank you enough. Kelly, Brooke, Shelby, Matt, Jessica, and Lauren, your smiles and encouragement carried me through more difficult days than you will ever know. Our time in Tennessee with you was a gift.

Ironically, Bennett's three private physical therapists were each named Kelly. He started off with Kelly in Virginia (who happened to be a dear friend of mine from Chantilly High School), moved on to Kelly in Tennessee, and ended with Kelly in Maryland. Each of these professionals aided us in keeping Bennett's physical health, safety, and daily tasks at an optimal level. The name Kelly comes from the Gaelic tradition and can mean "Warrior Maiden." It has always seemed fitting that Bennett's mother and his three main physical therapists would have that connotation, as wrestling with Bennett amidst his "moods" did indeed feel like a battle at times. Physical therapy is hard work, and these three Kellys were top notch professionals and true heroes.

To the staff at Stephen Knolls School who have loved a little boy from his first day in PEP at the age of three all the way up to high school, we are forever grateful. You are Bennett's second family, and the voices of Rob, the two Arlenes, Dan, and Jim bring an instant smile to Bennett's face. When Bennett boards his school bus each morning we are confident he will soon be greeted by a team ready to push him toward his greatest potential. Thank you does not seem adequate, but thank you nonetheless from the bottom of our hearts for educating our son with such passion and dedication.

To our community in Maryland, especially our neighbors and

friends, who care for our family on the good and bad days, walk alongside us in our challenges, and love all three of our kids unconditionally, we say thank you. Our Holy Redeemer school and church have blessed our family by giving us community in a way that we did not know was possible. We spent ten years in great isolation and then God led us to you. We are so grateful. And finally, to my WOWs, I cannot imagine life without your steadfast friendship, open arms, interceding prayer, and constant support.

To the Ezell Harding Christian School Community, Una Church of Christ, Fairfax Church of Christ, our childhood friends, Sunday school teachers, high school coaches, and our ACU professors and mentors — you directly helped shape us into who we are today. Thank you for all you poured into our hearts during our most formative years of development.

This book is also dedicated to both friends and strangers who have walked similar journeys ahead of us and behind us. Because of the love, sacrifice, and dedication that they have shown their children and the world, we are all stronger for it. We have gained fortitude by watching other parents care for their unique family situations, and frankly, it has made us feel less alone.

Couples who have inspired us along our journey include:

-Mike & Diane Cope (Megan) *Megan's Secrets*

-Gene & Ruth Ann Stallings (Johnny), *Another Season: A Coach's Story of Raising an Exceptional Son*

-Lon & Brenda Solomon (Jill) *Brokenness* (www.jillshouse.org)

-Katherine & Jay Wolf *Hope Heals* (www.hopeheals.com)

-Chad & Julia Veach (Georgia) *Unreasonable Hope*

-Jim & Jill Kelly (Hunter) *Without a Word*

-Mark & Muriel Forrest's Faith & Family Foundation (www.wheatlandfarm.org)

-Mark & Chelsea Jacobs (Gabe) (http://www.hischase.org/)

-My Life Speaks: Mike & Missy (Lane) (https://www.mylifes-peaks.com/)

Thank you to Laura and Tim for your steadfast friendship. All thanks to your special family, we met Mary Beth, Andy and Trevor — the team at Ballast Books who helped make this book happen. Many thanks to the Ballast team for believing in our story from the first paragraph sent, and leading us in our dream to share Bennett's story with the world.